W9-AXJ-537

Eye Movements
and Vision

Eye Movements
and Vision

by Alfred L. ~~Yarbus~~ Arbus

Institute for Problems of Information Transmission
Academy of Sciences of the USSR, Moscow

Translated from Russian by *Basil Haigh*
Cambridge, England

Translation Editor *Lorrin A. Riggs*
L. Herbert Ballou University Professor
Brown University, Providence, Rhode Island

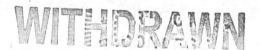

℗ PLENUM PRESS · NEW YORK · 1967

Al'fred Luk'yanovich Yarbus was born in Moscow in 1914. He was graduated from the Faculty of Physics of Moscow University in 1941 and was a scientific assistant at the Institute of Biophysics of the Academy of Sciences of the USSR until 1963. He is presently a senior scientist at the Institute for Problems of Information Transmission of the Academy. In 1964 he received the degree of Doctor of Biological Sciences for his work on "The Role of Eye Movements in Vision."

The original Russian text was published for the Institute of Information Transmission of the Academy of Sciences of the USSR by Nauka Press, Moscow, in 1965.

Альфред Лукьянович Ярбус

Роль движений глаз в процессе зрения

ROL' DVIZHENII GLAZ V PROTSESSE ZRENIYA

Library of Congress Catalog Card Number 66-19932

FOREWORD

This book is primarily a monograph describing the original re-
searches of the author. It is centered around a particular device,
originally described by Yarbus in 1956. This is an optical system in
miniature that can be attached by suction to the human eye. Many variations of the device—which we have called a "cap" for the sake of
brevity in this English edition—are described in detail in this book. One
form of the cap is particularly useful in the recording of eye movements; this permits the use of a plane mirror to achieve an optical
lever that writes a continuous record of eye position on the moving
film of a photokymograph. Of the greatest interest, however, are caps
that support an entire optical system. Attached by suction to the eyeball, such a system moves with it and hence confronts the observer
with a stationary visual field. The consequence is a rapid fading or
disappearance of the contours, colors, or other features of the field
that the author has explored. Thus the book is concerned not only with
the recording of eye movements in all their various forms, but also
with the consequences of eliminating the effects of eye movements on
visual perception.

A reading of this book cannot fail to impress one with the magnitude
of the whole research project. Yarbus has shown extraordinary skill
and ingenuity in the construction of delicate optics of sufficiently light
weight to be attached to the eye. The observer's task is not an easy
one. In most of the experiments the cornea is anesthetized, the lids
taped apart, and the subject trained to inhibit the natural tendency to
move the eyes about. These precautions are necessary in order to
keep the suction device from colliding with the lids and thus inflicting
injury on the device or on the eye itself. Although each experiment
was necessarily of limited duration, an impressive list of topics was
explored. The wide coverage, indeed, testifies to the author's acquaint-
ance with the significant problems of eye movements in their relation
to vision. In the field of psychology one would perhaps need to go back

v

to the nonsense-syllable experiments of Ebbinghaus to find an experimenter so enthusiastically exploiting a new experimental technique.

In all fairness one must recognize the limitations as well as the strengths of Yarbus' work. In fact, the recording of eye movements and the creation of a stabilized retinal image were achieved several years earlier, as Yarbus himself has acknowledged, in laboratories in America and England. Plastic contact lenses were used in those experiments. Poorly fitting lenses of this kind exhibit considerable slippage over the eyeball and hence may indeed be inferior to Yarbus' cap in experiments on eye movements and stabilized images, especially if loaded down with relatively heavy optical equipment. While the Yarbus cap has been used in at least one recent study in this country, the majority of investigators now rely upon tightly fitting contact lenses for their work. These have the advantage that they can be worn with comfort for the duration of an ordinary experiment without anesthesia, taping of lids, or the risk of corneal abrasion. Furthermore, recent evidence shows that when sufficient attention is given to the experimental conditions, the degree of slippage of a well-fitted contact lens is reduced to an amount too small to be of visual significance.

It may well turn out to be true that the Yarbus book has two lasting merits: First, as a stimulating account of what a single investigator can achieve on the basis of an ingenious experimental technique, and second, as a rich collection of ideas and observations of visual phenomena that deserve to be explored by future investigators.

                                                        Lorrin A. Riggs

Providence, R. I.
June 1967

PREFACE TO THE AMERICAN EDITION

The author is pleased to have the opportunity to acquaint the reader with the results of his work, the conclusions of which are of fundamental importance to the understanding of certain mechanisms of vision. The results of this work are largely due to an original technique, described fully in the book, employing suction devices, or "caps." In the author's opinion, this technique is suitable for use in studying a wide range of phenomena.

It would be a source of great satisfaction if this technique were to be adopted in the research laboratory and new and interesting results obtained by its use. It will, of course, be realized that experiments with "caps" are rather complex. They require great care and careful preparation in each case. Often the construction of the lenses and the accessories will have to be modified. A jeweller is required to make the very small details of the lenses and to assemble them, and of course this introduces considerable difficulty. However, the author knows of no easier method by which results similar to those described in this book can be obtained.

A. L. Yarbus

March 1967

PREFACE

This book deals with the perception of images which are strictly stationary relative to the retina, the principles governing human eye movements, and the study of their role in the process of vision.

The book is based on the results of the author's experimental investigations.

It is intended for students and researchers in the fields of biophysics, physiology, medicine, psychology, and branches of technology such as television, motion pictures, and apparatus construction. Much attention is devoted to the description of methods for recording eye movements and methods of producing images stationary relative to the retina. These methods may be of interest to many scientific workers.

The investigations were carried out in the laboratory of biophysics of vision of the Institute of Biophysics of the Academy of Sciences USSR, where they were discussed by all the staff. The author would like to emphasize particularly the help he has received for several years from N.D. Nyuberg and L.I. Seletskaya. The valuable advice of M. M. Bongard, A. L. Byzov, and M. S. Smirnov was frequently sought during these studies. Substantial technical assistance was given by V.I. Chernyshov, V. M. Timofeeva, P. N. Efimova, and I. N. Salina.

The author wishes to take this opportunity to express his sincere gratitude to all these colleagues and to the entire staff of the laboratory.

CONTENTS

INTRODUCTION

Recent developments have shown that our earlier ideas of the role of eye movement were considerably oversimplified. As the following facts will show, the subject as a whole is far more complex.

In man under natural conditions the retinal image is never stationary relative to the retina, and if a strictly stationary and unchanging retinal image is created artificially, the eye ceases to see. In other words, within any object of perception remaining strictly stationary relative to the retina and unchanging in time, after about 1-3 sec all visual contours disappear (the resolving power of the eye rapidly falls to zero).

It has long been known that an observer begins to see the blood vessels lying on the retina of his own eye when conditions are created in which the shadows of the vessels acquire some degree of mobility.

Experiments have shown that for the conditions of perception to be optimal, slight but not excessive continuous or interrupted movement of the retinal image over the retina is necessary, as a result of which the light acting on the receptors is constantly changing.

Electrophysiological studies have shown that as a rule impulses appear in the optic nerve of many animals only in response to a change in the light acting on the retina.

These facts have compelled a reassessment of the role of eye movements and have demonstrated that without an understanding of this role it is impossible to decipher the mechanisms of vision. For this reason it has become necessary, on the one hand, to study in detail the perception of images strictly stationary relative to the retina and changing in brightness or color and, on the other, to study the various forms of eye movements.

It was originally considered that the main function of the eye movements is to retain the object of perception in the visual field (to retain the element of the object important for perception in the fovea) and to change the points of fixation, thereby widening the total angle

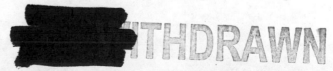

of view. Movements of the eyes preventing the disappearance of visual contours in the stationary object in the process of fixation now appear to be no less important.

The second chapter is the most important in the book. Concerned with the perception of objects stationary relative to the retina, it provides a new approach to certain sections of physiological optics, and helps to establish a number of connections and analogies between electrophysiological studies carried out on the retina in animals and studies of human vision.

The third chapter discusses the micromovements of the eyes accompanying the process of fixation directed towards a stationary object. This chapter explains how the micromovements of the eyes in ordinary conditions of perception prevent the disappearance of differences in the object during fixation. Changing the points of fixation, convergence and divergence of the optical axes, the pursuit of moving objects, and some cases of assessment of spatial relationships are accompanied by macromovements of the eyes.

Chapters IV through VII explain the role of, and the principles governing, macromovements of the eyes. Without an understanding of the role and knowledge of the principles of not only the micromovements, but also the macromovements of the eyes, the work of the retina cannot be completely understood. We shall refer to eye movements also when we speak about the structure of the eye and when we examine the special features of perception in man. For example, in phylogenesis the mobility of the head and eyes of some animals made possible the appearance of a fovea and introduced considerable refinement into the process of vision. These refinements are important because objects providing essential information are by no means uniformly distributed. Usually they are localized in small areas of the field of vision. In these circumstances the peripheral portion of the retina usually finds the object or element of an object which contains or may contain essential information, and consequently a process resembling reconnaissance takes place; this information is perceived and analyzed in greater detail by means of the foveal part of the retina, when directed towards the object.

The first chapter describes various methods of studying and recording eye movements, and methods for stabilizing the retinal image.

When understood, the role of eye movements and the principles governing these movements may help to solve many purely practical problems. Functional disturbances of the central nervous system are

often accompanied by disturbances of various eye movements. The centers controlling the eye movements and the pathways joining these centers to the eye muscles are located in various parts of the brain and are often adversely affected by pathological foci situated near these centers. The same is also true of disturbances in the working of the auxiliary systems closely connected with eye movements.

Any disturbances of the visual system in diseases of the central nervous system may help to determine both the character of the disease and the localization of the pathologic focus. However, it is not always simple to detect functional abnormality in an organ as complicated as the eye. It first becomes necessary to know what is normal. With respect to eye movements, this problem is far from solution. It is only in recent years that important data have been obtained in this field, and these data have not yet reached the attention of a wide range of readers for whom they would be of considerable interest. It should be emphasized here that disturbances of a patient's eye movement can be recorded objectively, and that this procedure is particularly applicable for diagnostic purposes.

Knowledge of the principles governing eye movement in the normal subject may be useful also in ophthalmology. Unfortunately, no systematic records of eye movements have yet been made in the various forms of strabismus, paralyses, and pareses of the eye muscles. It is by no means impossible, for example, that such records could be used to diagnose and to distinguish objectively the treatable and un- treatable forms of strabismus.

Familiarity with the perception of objects stationary relative to the retina and changing in color or brightness undoubtedly is useful to the neurologist and ophthalmologist. Disturbances of this perception in patients may also give useful information regarding the character of a disease of the central nervous system or of the eye.

In many cases when an investigator is interested in the problem of perception of complex objects (in normal and pathologic conditions), records of the eye movements would be valuable. In these circum- stances, by using such records it would be easy to determine the order in which an object was examined, what elements were fixated by the subject, how often and for how long a particular element was fixated, and so on. Records of eye movements illustrate the course of the process of perception.

Knowledge of the principles governing eye movements and the properties of perception of images stationary relative to the retina may be used (and sometimes is used) in motion pictures and television, in apparatus construction, for the rational arrangement of instruments on panels, for evaluating the possibilities of perception in complex conditions, and so on.

Chapter I

METHODS

1. ELEMENTARY FACTS CONCERNING THE STRUCTURE OF THE HUMAN EYE*

The outer layer of the eye (Fig. 1) is formed of a tough membrane, the sclera, consisting of firm connective tissue continuous in its anterior part with a transparent membrane, the cornea. The sclera enables the eye to maintain a constant shape and protects its contents. The same function is served by the cornea, which is also part of the dioptric apparatus of the eye. The membranes of the eye are under a certain intraocular pressure. The normal intraocular pressure lies within the limits of 15–30 mm Hg.

The dioptric apparatus of the eye, which takes part in the formation of an image on its inner surface, consists of the cornea, the biconvex transparent lens, the transparent aqueous humor, and the transparent vitreous, filling the eye. This apparatus also includes the ciliary body, which allows changes to be made (by means of the ciliary muscle) in the curvature of the lens surfaces (accommodation) and the iris, which modifies the diameter of the pupil (the aperture of the diaphragm). Accommodation permits the image to be sharply focused. A change in the size of the pupil leads to changes in the retinal illuminance and the depth of focus of the optical system. The optical system gives an inverted real image of objects in front of the eye.

The diameter of the average eye in all meridians is approximately 24 mm.

Beneath the sclera lies the vascular membrane, consisting of a network of blood vessels supplying the eye. Next to the inner surface of the vascular membrane lies the pigmented epithelium, containing

---

*Detailed information concerning the structure and function of the eye can be found in the works of Averbakh (1940), Kravkov (1950), Tonkov (1946), and Polyak (1941).

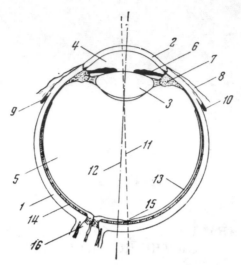

Fig. 1. Scheme of a horizontal section of the human right eye. 1) Sclera; 2) cornea; 3) lens; 4) anterior chamber of the eye; 5) vitreous; 6) iris; 7) ciliary muscle; 8) conjunctiva; 9) point of attachment of medial rectus muscle; 10) point of attachment of lateral rectus muscle; 11) visual axis of the eye; 12) optical axis of eye; 13) retina; 14) vascular membrane; 15) fovea centralis; 16) optic nerve.

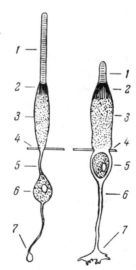

Fig. 2. Rods and cones of the retina. Left, a rod: 1) outer segment; 2) ellipsoid; 3) inner segment; 4) outer limiting membrane; 5) rod fiber; 6) nucleus; 7) terminal bouton. Right, a cone: 1) outer segment; 2) ellipsoid; 3) inner segment; 4) outer limiting membrane; 5) nucleus; 6) cone fiber; 7) cone foot-plate (Averbakh, 1940).

a dark pigment. Beyond the layer of pigmented epithelium is the innermost layer which directly receives the photic stimuli, the retina. Schematically, the retina can be divided into two zones: a photosensitive zone facing the vascular membrane, and a neural zone, facing the vitreous. The thickness of the retina in its central part, the macula lutea, is about 0.1 mm.

The photosensitive cells of the retina (receptors) are the rods and cones (Fig. 2). The rods are much more sensitive to light than the cones. At very low levels of illumination only the rods function, and they are associated with the mechanism of twilight vision. The rods contain a photosensitive pigment with a maximum spectral sensitivity at a wavelength of 510 mμ. The cones contain three photosensitive pigments with spectral sensitivity maxima at wavelengths of 440, 540, and 590 mμ (Fig. 3). The cones are associated with the mechanism of color vision.

The point of entry of the optic nerve into the eye has no rods or cones. We cannot see with this part of the retina, and it is therefore called the blind spot. The point of clearest vision is the macula lutea. It lies on the temporal side, slightly above the point of entry of the optic nerve (Fig. 1). The macula lutea is yellow and occupied mainly by cones. The angular dimension of the macula lutea is approximately 6-7°. Within the macula lutea lies the fovea centralis, the part of the retina with the highest resolving power. The diameter of the fovea centralis is about 0.4 mm, i.e., about 1.3°. The middle part of the fovea centralis (the foveola) is pigmented less than the other parts of the macula lutea. The fovea centralis is slightly displaced from the optical axis of the eye.

In the human retina there are about 130 million rods and about 7 million cones. The distribution of the rods and cones in the retina is indicated in Figs. 4 and 5. The diameter of the inner segment of

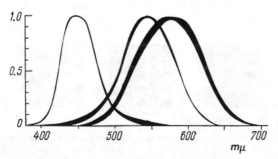

Fig. 3. Curves of sensitivity of human daylight receptors—cones (Bongard and Smirnov, 1955).

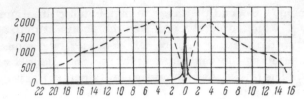

Fig. 4. Distribution of rods and cones in the retina. Abscissa—the distance (in mm) from the middle of the fovea centralis (the foveola) along the horizontal section of the right eye. Ordinate—the number of hundreds of rods and cones per mm^2. The broken line represents rods and the solid line cones (Oesterberg, 1935).

the rod is about 0.002 mm. The diameter of the inner segment of the cones varies with the position in the retina from approximately 0.002 to 0.007 mm. The cones in the central part of the retina, where the distance between the centers of the cones is about 0.0025 mm (0.5 minute of angle), are longer and thinner than in the peripheral part. The resolving power of the eye is maximal at the fovea centralis and gradually diminishes towards the periphery. The relative visual acuity in relation to the position of the image on the retina is shown in Fig. 6.

The structure of the retina is very complex (Fig. 7). Morphologists (Polyak, 1941) have distinguished the following 10 layers in the retina: 1, the pigmented epithelium; 2, the layer of outer and inner segments of rods and cones; 3, the outer limiting membrane, intersected by the rods and cones; 4, the outer nuclear layer containing the nuclei and fibers of the rods and cones; 5, the outer plexiform layer, formed by a plexus of endings of the photoreceptors with the fibers of neurons of the next layer; 6, the inner nuclear layer of bipolar cells, horizontal and amacrine; 7, the inner plexiform layer, consisting of a plexus of endings of the neurons of layer 6 with the endings of the ganglion cells; 8, the layer of ganglion cells; 9, the layer of fibers of the optic nerve; and 10, the inner limiting membrane. The bipolar cells are of several types, differing in morphological structure and in mode of communica-

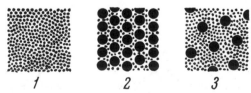

Fig. 5. Relative distribution of rods and cones in the retina. 1) Mosaic of cones in the center of the fovea; 2) rods (small dots) and cones (large dots) 0.8 mm from the center of the fovea; 3) rods and cones 3 mm from the center of the fovea (Averbakh, 1940).

tion with other neurons. The same is true of the ganglion cells. The final centers of vision are the occipital lobes of the cerebral cortex, on both lips of the calcarine fissure.

The part of the optic pathway from the eye to the chiasma (the point of partial decussation of the optic nerves) is called the optic nerve. The optic nerve, about 5 cm long and about 4 mm^2 in cross section consists of approximately 1 million nerve fibers. There are, on the average, about 150 rods and cones to each fiber. At the chiasma the optic nerve divides into two parts (Fig. 8). The fibers running from the nasal half of the retina proceed to the opposite cerebral hemisphere; fibers arising from the temporal half of the retina proceed to the hemisphere on the same side. Therefore there is an incomplete decussation of the optic nerves in the chiasma. The optic nerve fibers forming the optic tract then run to the subcortical visual centers (the pulvinar of the thalamus, the anterior colliculi, the lateral geniculate body). From the intermediate centers, nerve fibers known as Gratiolet's fibers run to the terminal visual centers. After reaching the geniculate body, some fibers continue to the temporal region of the brain. Injuries to the brain and corresponding disturbances of the visual fields of the eye have demonstrated the connections between various parts of the retina and the cerebral cortex. This projection of the retina on the cortex is illustrated in Fig. 9.

The position of the eyes in the orbits is shown schematically in Fig. 10. Under normal conditions eye movements cause practically no displacement of the center of the eye relative to the orbit. All movements of the eye amount to its rotation about a certain center lying inside the eye on the optical axis. The distance between the

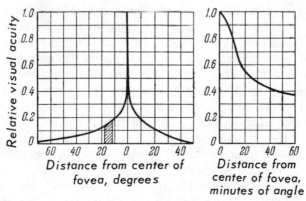

Fig. 6. Relative visual acuity depending on the position of the retinal image of the retina (Jones and Higgins, 1947).

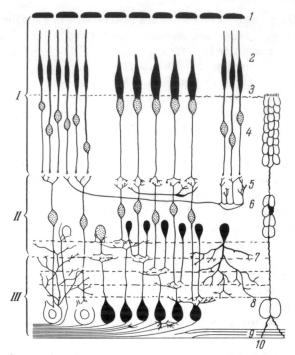

Fig. 7. Scheme showing the structure of the retina. I, II, and III. First, second, and third
neurons. A sustentacular fiber of Müller is shown on the right (Kravkov, 1950).

apex of the cornea and the center of rotation of the eye is approximately
14.5 mm. Rotation of the eye around this center is performed by three
pairs of muscles (Fig. 11). These muscles (named in accordance with
their position) are: the lateral and medial rectus muscles; the superior
and inferior rectus muscles; and the superior and inferior oblique
muscles. The four rectus muscles arise by tendons in the depths of
the orbit. They are all attached to the eye several millimeters from
the edge of the cornea. The inferior oblique muscle runs from the
anterior part of the orbit laterally and winds around the eye to which
it is attached posteriorly. The superior oblique muscle arises in the
depth of the orbit, runs forward, passing over a special pulley, turns
posteriorly and laterally, and is attached to the postero-superior part
of the eye. The intermediate space between the eye and its orbit is
filled with orbital fat, on which the eye rests. In addition, the eye is
maintained in position by special ligaments.

The work of the muscles during rotation of the eye is fairly
complex. The action of the individual eye muscles is shown schematically in Fig. 12. Of all the voluntary muscles in the body, the eye

muscles possess the thinnest fibers. The eye muscles are very profusely innervated by motor and sensory nerve fibers (Duke-Elder, 1932; Fulton, 1943). The eye muscles are innervated by the oculo-motor, trochlear, and abducens nerves. The trochlear nerve supplies the superior oblique muscle and the abducens nerve the lateral rectus. The oculomotor nerve innervates all the other muscles of the eye, including the ciliary muscle and the muscles responsible for changing the size of the pupil. All these nerves arise in the lower part of the brain in the floor of the 4th ventricle, in the region of the corpora quadrigemina, pons, and medulla.

2. STUDY OF EYE MOVEMENTS BY MEANS OF AFTER-IMAGES

Modern methods of recording eye movements and of creating a stabilized retinal image are by no means perfect. Frequently, when new methods are being developed, long established methods are used. In some cases, even complicated problems can be solved by the use of "forgotten" techniques. This suggests that a short historical review of methods related to this theme would be worth while.

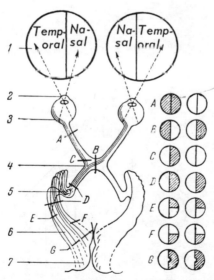

Fig. 8. Scheme showing the optic pathways and centers. 1) Field of vision; 2) cornea; 3) retina; 4) chiasma; 5) subcortical visual centers; 6) Gratiolet's fibers; 7) visual cortex. Defects arising in the visual field after injuries to the optic pathways are indicated on the right. The blind area in the visual field is shaded. The point of injury is denoted by a stroke and letter on the figure on the left (Kravkov, 1950).

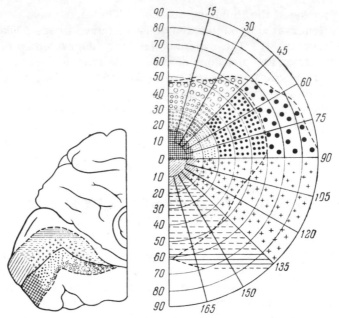

Fig. 9. Projection of visual field on the cerebral cortex. The numbers denote degrees (Holmes, 1918).

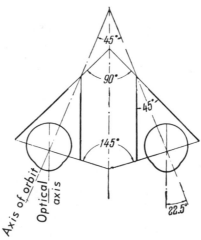

Fig. 10. Scheme showing the positions of the eyes in the orbits (Duke–Elder, 1932).

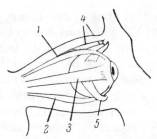

Fig. 11. Scheme showing the muscles of the eye. 1) Superior rectus muscle; 2) inferior rectus muscle; 3) lateral rectus muscle (medial rectus lies symmetrically opposite but cannot be seen on the drawing); 4) superior oblique muscle; 5) inferior oblique muscle.

Several experimenters (Dodge, 1907; Helmholtz, 1925; Duke-Elder, 1932; Barlow, 1952; and others) have studied the character of eye movements by the use of after-images. Eye movements were studied in the process of fixation, in the process of changing points of fixation, and during examination of complex objects. With the introduction of modern flash lamps, this method of producing after-images has become much more refined. The blinding brightness and short duration of the flash (less than 0.001 sec) make it possible to produce long after-images of great sharpness.

Let us examine a well known method of observing the movement of the eye itself in the process of fixation. The experimenter produces a clear after-image (reference mark) projected on the fovea and shaped like a cross, a line, or a small triangle. The observer then fixates on a point on a screen, which is either a sheet of graph paper or paper on which a grid has been drawn During fixation, the observer at the same time watches the movement of the reference mark relative to the point of fixation and to the grid of the screen and notes the trajectory followed by the mark during a particular period of time.

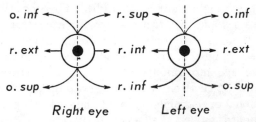

Fig. 12. Direction of action of the individual eye muscles. Broken line—vertical meridian of the eye; black circle—pupil; r. ext.—lateral rectus muscle; r. int.—medial rectus muscle; r. sup.—superior rectus muscle; r. inf.—inferior rectus muscle; o. sup.—superior oblique muscle; o. inf.—inferior oblique muscle (Kravkov, 1950).

Since the after-image is strictly stationary relative to the retina, the apparent movement of this image on the screen corresponds directly to the movements of the eye. Knowing the distance between the eye and screen, it is easy to calculate the size of the division on the grid of the screen in angular values, and to determine the eye movements performed during fixation with rough accuracy. In this case the sharpness of the after-image is very important. The smaller the reference mark and the sharper it appears to the eye, obviously the greater the accuracy with which its movement on the screen can be determined.

Another method of studying eye movements in the process of fixation is as follows. The observer fixates on a point placed at the center of a narrow slit. A flash lamp is placed behind each half of the slit. The flash lamps are switched on consecutively at a predetermined interval, equal to some fraction of a second. In these circumstances after-images appear from each half of the slit. As a result of the eye movements in the interval between two flashes, the two halves of the after-image usually appear displaced relative to each other. From the magnitude of this displacement, the experimenter can judge the magnitude and character of the eye movement during fixation.

Observations on the large eye movements during examination of an object can be conveniently made by means of an after-image in the shape of a circle projected on the fovea. Knowing the angular size of the circle, and memorizing its position on the object during perception, the observer can judge approximately with which parts of the retina he looks at a particular element of the object and what information is obtained in this process.

The general character of eye movements during examination of stationary objects, the jerkiness of these movements in particular, has been studied in the past (Landolt, 1891) as follows. The observer sits in a dark room and a weakly illuminated object is placed in his field of vision, while against this background, or alongside it, is placed a small but very bright source of light. The observer looks at the object or traces its outline with his eye for a certain period of time, after which the light is switched off. From the series of after-images produced by the bright source of light, the observer can judge the character of the eye movements. Each separate after-image corresponds to a point of fixation; each interval between two neighboring points of fixation corresponds to a change of the points of fixation.

Eye movements during a change in points of fixation have been studied by several authors (Lamansky, 1869; Cobb and Moss, 1925) by means of a bright flashing source of light. The light source, flashing at a frequency of several hundred cycles per second was placed between two points of fixation. During change in the points of fixation, as a result of the flashes of the source of light and the eye movements, a series of images of the source of light was obtained on the retina; subsequently, after the light was extinguished, these were perceived by the observer as a chain of after-images. Since the observer always knew the flash frequency, the number of after-images and the angle between the points of fixation, he could determine the time of alternation of the points of fixation.

Several authors (Loring, 1915) also used after-images to find rotary movement of the eye around the optical axis. Here, the after-image (a cross) was projected by the observer on a screen with a grid of horizontal and vertical lines. The observer chose the point of fixation and put his head in a position in which the lines of the cross were parallel to the lines of the grid. He then performed a movement with his eye and remembered when and approximately at which angle the lines of the cross changed their direction relative to the grid on the screen. The visible rotation of the cross relative to its own center corresponded to the rotation of the eye relative to the axis of vision.

If an observer looks at a very bright white field through a red filter, and the red filter is then changed for a violet (or the whole procedure is performed in the opposite order), each time, shortly after the change of filter, he can see the fovea of the opposite eye in the form of a tiny star. By fixating on a point on the bright field and memorizing the movement of the fovea, in these circumstances, the observer can obtain some idea of the eye movements during fixation.

As a result of adaptation, prolonged fixation on any object composed of contrasting elements separated by sharp boundaries leads to appreciable diminution of the sharpness of the visible differences in color between the elements. Under these circumstances, however, as a result of small eye movements, sharp bands appear at the border between the elements of the object. From the way in which these bands appear and from their width, some idea may also be obtained of the eye movements during fixation.

Today eye movements are rarely studied by means of after-images because more refined methods have been developed. This does not mean, however, that after-images have now served their purpose as a method of investigation and will never again be used in laboratory practice. Let me give a few examples.

First, after-images may be used whenever an experimenter is interested in the perception of objects stationary relative to the retina (after-images are always stationary relative to the retina), for example, the perception of the shape or proportions of an object in

conditions when the subject cannot use eye movement, or the perception
of optical illusions in the same conditions, and so on.

If an intracranial tumor has deprived a patient of half his field of
vision (hemianopsia), several authors have suggested that a "pseudo-
fovea" may appear within the functioning part of the retina of each eye.
To localize this point, and to trace its evolution, it is best to use
after-images.   An experiment in this case could be conceived as
follows: the patient is asked to fixate on the center of a geometrical
figure (for example, several concentric circles). Next, by means of
a flash lamp the patient is made to develop an after-image of this
shape. Naturally, the patient sees only part of the shape as the after-
image—the part on the functioning half of the retina at the time of
fixation on the center of the figure. If the patient fixated by the use of
the pseudo-fovea, this part would be greater than half and the corresponding difference (the difference between the visible part and half
the figure, measured in angular units) would show how far the pseudo-
fovea was shifted relative to the center of the retina.

The apparent size of the after-image, like the apparent size of the
real object, is determined by several factors, and above all by the size
of the retinal image. It changes appreciably with a change in convergence and accommodation, and with considerable deflection of the
gaze up or down. Since the retinal image corresponding to the after-
image remains strictly unchanged the whole time, the after-image is
a convenient test for the influence of various factors accompanying
perception and changing the apparent size.

3. DETERMINING THE MAGNITUDE OF INVOLUNTARY EYE MOVEMENTS DURING THE PERCEPTION OF SMALL OBJECTS

When examining an object, determining its proportions, counting
the elements of an object, and so on, we usually use eye movements
and voluntarily change the points of fixation. It has been found that
if an observer cannot use voluntary eye movements, the solution of
certain problems of perception (determination of proportions, comparison of areas, counting large numbers of small elements, and so
on) becomes difficult, even when the corresponding retinal image is
completely within the fovea and, consequently, all elements of the
object are clearly seen. There are a number of methods by which eye
movements can be excluded artificially during perception. Under
certain conditions, a similar situation may even arise in a normal
subject.   During fixation directed towards a stationary object, the

human eyes involuntarily perform small, jerky movements. If the angular dimensions of the object are smaller than these movements, the observer cannot make out the various elements separately, using voluntary eye movements. The solution of these problems under such conditions presents considerable difficulties. The fact that such difficulties can arise has been used by several workers to determine the magnitude of the involuntary eye movements during fixation. Landolt (1891), in an attempt to determine the smallest angle of the voluntary eye movement, instructed a subject to count a number of vertical lines forming a regular series. The lines were placed far enough away from the subject so that he could not count them but near enough so that be could clearly distinguish them. Landolt believed that the difficulty experienced by the subject in counting the lines corresponded to a situation in which voluntary eye movements were impossible. This method cannot, of course, compete with modern methods allowing eye movements to be recorded objectively.

4. EARLY METHODS OF STUDYING PERCEPTION OF OBJECTS STATIONARY RELATIVE TO THE RETINA

In 1804, Troxler found that objects visible to the periphery of the eye disappear during careful fixation on a certain point. This phenomenon was called Troxler's effect (Claıke, 1960). The first correct interpretation of this effect was evidently given by Adrian (1928). By using the results of electrophysiology (in most animals, impulses appear in the optic nerve only in response to a change in the light acting on the retina), Adrian suggested that the human eye also stops working under conditions where the retinal image is unchanged and stationary. Adrian himself tried by very careful fixation to obtain disappearance of visible differences within an object, on one point of which he fixated. In certain conditions he could do this for a short time, but these experiments were not very convincing. However, there are several well known methods by which this property of human vision may be illustrated.

We know that large blood vessels run along the inner surface of the retina. Although these are not usually seen, conditions can easily be created in which the shadows of these vessels become visible on the retina. If these shadows continually change their size or position, they will be continually and clearly seen by the observer. Of the experiments of this series, the following is the most effective procedure.

An observer in a dark room takes a bright-point source of light in, let us say, his right hand and holds it in front of him below the level of the eyes. With his left hand, he covers his left eye and with his right eye he looks at a large dark screen or at the wall. The observer then makes a continuous waving movement with his right hand during which the moving source of light is always visible to the eye at the extreme periphery of the retina. Under these conditions sharp outlines of the eye vessels appear, and they seem to the observer to be projected on the screen. As soon as the observer stops moving the source of light (i.e., the movement of the shadows of the vessels), the vessels disappear within 1-2 seconds, but reappear when movement of the light source is resumed.

I will mention one further method by which an observer can see the vessels of his eye. An opaque diaphragm with a very small aperture (for example, a piece of black paper pierced by a fine needle) is placed in front of the eye, near the cornea. The observer looks through the aperture at a bright screen and at the same time gives the diaphragm an oscillatory movement of small amplitude. The movement of the aperture in front of the pupil causes excursions of the rays of light over the retina, and this in turn causes movement of the shadows of the vessels and their appearance in the field of vision. The vessels are seen much better if the pupil is artificially dilated before the experiment.

Even with the most careful fixation on a point, it is impossible to obtain the complete disappearance of the visual contours, usually because of involuntary movements of the eyes and head. However, there is one very simple experiment which demonstrates this possibility. The observer sits on a chair near a lamp and sticks a few small pieces of paper of different colors to the right half of his nose, to that part which can easily be seen with the right eye. He then rests his elbows on the chair arms, covers the left eye with the left hand, and uses the right hand as a chin rest. He then chooses a point of fixation on the chair so that it lies next to the pieces of colored paper sticking to his nose. At a certain moment, after a short period of fixation, the visible part of the nose and the brightly illuminated pieces of paper completely lose their color and appear as a uniform dark grey field. A slight movement of the eye instantaneously restores the disappearing differences. The relative ease with which in this case success can be obtained is explained by the fact that, because of the closeness of the pieces of paper to the eye, the retinal image is out of focus, and its outlines are not sharp. Under these conditions, small movements of the eyes are less important. The methods described can supply valuable illustrations when demonstrating the work of the eye.

5. STUDY OF EYE MOVEMENTS BY VISUAL OBSERVATION

A general idea of the character of the eye movements can be obtained by direct visual observation of the eye. Some authors (Javal, 1879) used a mirror for this purpose. Observations were made on the image of the eye in a mirror. The experimenter stood behind the subject and did not distract him during the experiment. However, with the unaided eye, the experimenter could observe only large movements. Rotation of the eye through 1°, and the corresponding movement of the retina through 0.2 mm could not be noticed by the experimenter. Later optical instruments were used to provide a magnified image of the eye, or of part of it, thus increasing the accuracy of the method. Lenses giving the required magnification were used in the study of relatively large eye movements (Newhall, 1928), and a microscope was used in the study of small eye movements or movements during fixation (Gassovskii and Nikol'skaya, 1941). In the second case the experimenter made observations with the microscope on the movement of a bifurcation of the blood vessels.

Since the ready-made optical instruments were not always satisfactory for these purposes, specially designed instruments were created. Some authors (George, Toren, and Löwell, 1923; Park and Park, 1933) studied the position of the center of rotation of the eye in relation to the direction of fixation. In this work, observations were made on the apex of the cornea by means of special optical instruments. The center of rotation of the eye did not remain strictly stationary relative to the eye, for during rotation of the eye the apex of the cornea moved over a surface slightly different from that of a sphere. Given this difference for many directions of fixation, it was relatively easy to determine the geometrical localization of the points, from which the position of the corresponding centers of rotation could be determined. Park (1936a, 1936b) and Park and Park (1940) used a special goniometer to study eye movements during fixation. The eye movements were studied in connection with the movement of the lens. In the opinion of these authors, fixation on a point is accompanied by continuous movement of the eye and lens. Peckham (1934) and Ogle, Mussey, and Prangen (1949) used a stereoscope and telescopes to study changes in convergence during fixation on an object.

Because of the creation of specially devised optical instruments the method of visual observations is still suitable for the study of certain types of eye movement today. However, the newer methods, which provide more objective records, have proved more accurate and therefore preferable.

6. MECHANICAL RECORDING OF EYE MOVEMENTS

In the past several authors have used methods by which the connection between the eye and the recording instrument was mechanical. Three types of these methods are known.

The first type utilized the convexity of the cornea; the movement of the cornea (like the cam on a camshaft) was transmitted by a lever and balance arm. The fulcrum in which the lever rotated was fixed to the subject's head. One polished end of the lever, under slight pressure, touched the anesthetized surface of the eye. The other end made the record on a moving paper tape. The subject's head was usually held in a headrest. This method was used by Ohm (1914, 1916, 1928) and Cords (1927).

In the second type, the convexity of the cornea again was used, but this time the movement was transmitted, not to a lever, but to an elastic rubber balloon filled with air. The balloon was fixed so that it pressed lightly against the anesthetized surface of the eye. Movement of the eye altered the pressure inside the balloon, and this change was transmitted along a thin tube to the recording system.

In the third type of method, small cups resembling contact lenses were used. In the center of the cup was an aperture or window through which the subject looked at the object to be perceived. The cup was affixed to the anesthetized eye like a contact lens. A lever or thread was attached to the cup by means of which the eye movements were transmitted to the recording system. Delabarre (1898) and Huey (1898, 1900) used cups made of plaster of Paris, while Orschansky (1899) used aluminum cups. In some experiments Orschansky fixed a small mirror to the cup; he was evidently the first to use a beam of light reflected and projected on a screen to study eye movements.

Today mechanical methods of recording eye movements are outmoded. Their accuracy is low, and they are more complicated than many modern methods.

7. RECORDING EYE MOVEMENTS BY A REFLECTED
BEAM OF LIGHT

By some means or other a plane mirror is affixed to the subject's eye. A beam of light is transmitted to the mirror from a source whose diaphragm may contain a narrow slit or a small hole. The reflected beam is directed to photosensitive material and focused on it in the form of a bright narrow band (if the record is made on the moving photosensitive tape of a photokymograph). The reflected light beam reproduces the eye movements and records them on photosensitive material. During the experiment the subject's head is held in a head-rest. The lids of the anesthetized eye are taped open with strips of adhesive plaster, or the experimenter holds them open with his hands.

Several methods are known for affixing a mirror to the eye. Marx and Trendelenburg (1911) glued the mirror to an aluminum cup resembling a contact lens. The cup together with the mirror was attached to the eye like a contact lens. Dohlman (1925) used a rubber cup instead of an aluminum one, while Adler and Fliegelman (1934) attached the mirror directly to the sclera of the eye. Riggs and Ratliff (1949, 1950, 1951) used contact lenses to which mirrors were attached. In this case there was no need to anesthetize the eye. More recently, contact lenses have been used by many workers (Ginsborg, 1952; Ditchburn and Ginsborg, 1953; Riggs, Armington, and Ratliff, 1954; Nachmias, 1959, 1960; Krauskopf, Cornsweet, and Riggs, 1960; Riggs and Niehl, 1960; and others). Contact lenses have been used for monocular and binocular records, and other simple devices, have made possible the simultaneous recording of the vertical and horizontal components of eye movements. Moreover, the contact lens began to be used as a base unit to which other devices required for solving particular experimental problems or for the development of new techniques were affixed instead of the mirror. Finally, instead of contact lenses, the present author has used small rubber suction cups with mirrors which, by virtue of their very small mass, provided a firm link between the mirror and the eye (Yarbus, 1954). A full description of this method is given below.

The method of recording eye movements by a reflected beam of light is the most sensitive of any presently known method. Its great drawback is that it cannot be used when for some reason no apparatus of any kind can be affixed to the subject's eye. Another disadvantage of the method is the creation of distortion in the records (distortion during recording with a reflected beam of light will be considered in detail later). On the question of contact lenses it should be noted that although in many cases they are very convenient and in fact irreplaceable, they possess two important disadvantages. The contact lens has a definite mass which, when affixed to the eye, changes its moment of inertia considerably. This modifies eye movements taking place with high acceleration (e.g., voluntary saccadic movements and tremor movements). The second important disadvantage of the ordinary

contact lens is that it is not firmly joined to the eye. During a fast
movement, the contact lens is displaced very slightly, sliding over the
eye surface.

8. STUDY OF EYE MOVEMENTS BY STILL AND MOTION-PICTURE PHOTOGRAPHY

Many authors have used motion-picture and still photography to
study eye movements. In methods of this type, the eye movements
were judged from the consecutive movement of images of a particular
element of the eye relative to a reference point that was firmly affixed to the subject's head. In some methods in which good fixation
of the head was achieved, the initial position of the eye itself was taken
as the point of reference.

Dodge and Cline (1901) were evidently the first to make photographic
studies of the eye in movement. They photographed the eyes on a still
photographic plate and obtained a series of images of the eye displaced
relative to each other and corresponding to a condition of individual
fixations. Analysis of this film gave an idea of the character of the
eye movements.

A more refined method was used by Judd, McAllister, and Steele
(1905). They took sequential photographs (about nine frames per second) of the eye and part of the face. A small spot of Chinese white
was placed on the cornea. The subject's head was held in a headrest,
and two small shining balls were affixed to it; since these fell within the
exposure field of the objective lens, they were photographed in each
frame and could be used as the origin of the coordinates. The position
of the white spot relative to this origin of the coordinates was determined in each frame and after suitable analysis of all the frames a
descriptive account of the eye movements was obtained.

Karslake (1940) made motion pictures of the image of the eye in a
semitransparent mirror, through which the subject looked at the
object of perception. In this method the apparatus was behind the
subject and did not distract him during the experiment.

Barlow (1952) used the following method. A very small drop of
mercury was placed on the subject's cornea. A second drop was placed
on the forehead. By means of a microscope the images of the two
drops were projected and recorded on a moving film. The combined
movements of eye and head were judged from the record of the movements of the drop placed on the cornea. The movements of the head
were judged from the record of the movements of the drop on the

forehead. During the experiment the subject's head was fixed, which restricted its movement.

Higgins and Stultz (1953), in order to study eye movements during fixation, photographed a magnified image of a blood vessel of the sclera on a moving film. The optical system of the apparatus magnified the vessel 26 times, and the vessel was chosen so that its image was perpendicular to the aperture of the apparatus. The part of the sclera containing the vessel to be photographed was illuminated with ultraviolet light. For the control observations of the head movement, a marker fixed to the subject's nose was recorded at the same time. Haberich and Fischer (1958) studied the blinking movements of the eye during alternation of the points of fixation by means of a device called a time lens. In one second the time lens gave 64 images of the eye on a film. The turning movements of the head were recorded simultaneously on the film. A. R. Shakhnovich and V. R. Shakhnovich (1961) described an apparatus in which images of both the subject's eyes were projected in the plane of the aperture of a photokymograph. A compensating prism rotated in front of this aperture and displaced the image in a direction perpendicular to the aperture. In these conditions scanning of the pupil takes place and an impression of its diameter is obtained on the film. Both the vertical and horizontal diameters of each pupil may be projected in the plane of the aperture of the optic system. Both components (vertical and horizontal) of the movement of each eye are recorded on the film. The accuracy of the method is low, and it is therefore suitable for recording the large movements of the eyes have to be recorded. Their main disadvantage the size of the pupil is recorded at the same time.

In evaluating methods of recording eye movements based on still and motion-picture photography, it must be remembered that these methods can be used successfully in many cases when the large movements of the eyes have to be recorded. Their main disadvantage is the relatively laborious method of analysis of the records required.

9. RECORDING THE CORNEAL BRIGHT SPOT

The radius of curvature of the cornea is approximately 8 mm, and that of the eye about 12 mm. The center of curvature of the cornea is displaced 3-5 mm relative to the center of rotation of the eye. The cornea, like the convex surface of a lens, reflects part of the light falling on its surface as the corneal reflex (the sparkle of the eyes). Since the center of rotation of the eye and the center of curvature of the cornea do not coincide, the angle at which a stationary source of light is reflected in the cornea changes during a movement of the eye so that the corneal reflex moves when the eye moves. Several authors have used the corneal reflex to study eye movements. This method appeared very tempting—eye movements could be studied without touching the eye itself. However, every experimenter has become clearly aware of the drawbacks of this method. Very small movements of the reflex always take place against the background of head movements and are added to them, so that the accuracy of the records is considerably reduced. In almost every variant of the method, very reliable fixation of the subject's head or rigid fixation of optical instruments to it is required, in order to avoid artifacts caused by movements of the head. In addition, displacements of the reflex are sometimes caused by changes in the thickness of the layer of tear fluid covering the cornea, especially near the lids. Finally, the relationship between the eye movement and the movement of the reflex has been found to be complicated.

The first authors who photographed the corneal reflex to study eye movements were Dodge and Cline (1901) and Stratton (1902, 1906). Dodge (1907) recorded the movements of the reflex on a falling photographic plate. He studied the eye movements in the process of fixation, pursuit, and reading. Stratton recorded the movements of the reflex on a stationary photographic plate when the subject examined complicated geometrical figures. The methods of photography of the corneal reflexes were subsequently improved, and special apparatus was introduced. Particular attention was paid to the creation of apparatuses designed to record the reflexes of both eyes during reading (Tinker, 1931; Taylor, 1937). Apparatuses were also devised to allow simultaneous records to be made of the vertical and horizontal movements of the reflex (Weaver, 1931; Clark, 1934). Two variants of the apparatus specially designed for studying eye movements during fixation were developed by Hartridge and Thomson (1948). To avoid the influence of head movements on the records, these authors constructed a special alabaster cap to which the light source, the point of fixation, and some optical instruments were fixed. The cap was secured firmly to the subject's head. The light source and the corneal reflex were photographed simultaneously by a motion-picture camera with a frequency of 60 frames per second. In the other, more refined variant of the method, the subject held between his teeth a special plate fixed to the optical system during the experiment. The optical system rotated freely in all directions and did not encumber the subject's head.

Besides these photographic methods, Lord and Wright have recently developed a photoelectric method of recording the movements of the corneal reflex (Lord, 1948, 1951, 1952a, 1952b; Lord and Wright, 1948, 1949). This method has been used mainly to study eye movements during fixation. These authors claim that a rotary movement of the eye amounting to only one minute of angle can be recorded by means of this method. In their experiments, the subject lay on his back, his head strapped to a special headrest. The subject held between his teeth a plate firmly fixed to the headrest. A beam of ultraviolet light with a wavelength of 365 mμ was thrown on the cornea, reflected from it, and when it fell on a semitransparent aluminized mirror, separated into two parts. One part of the beam was directed towards the edge of a vertical screen and the other part to the edge of a horizontal screen. Behind each screen and partly covered by it was a photoelectric cell. One photoelectric cell detected the changes in the horizontal component and the other the changes in the vertical component of the movements of the corneal reflex. The current from the photoelectric cells was fed into a DC amplifier and then into a cathode-ray oscilloscope. Mackworth and Mackworth (1958) used a television technique to record eye movements. The image of the object of perception and the corneal reflex, magnified 100 times, were transmitted to the screen of a television tube and coupled in such a way that the position of the reflex on the object corresponded to the point of fixation. According to these authors, this method allowed the eye movement to be recorded with an accuracy of up to 1-2°.

All the methods based on recording the corneal reflex can be used only to record relatively large movements of the eyes.

10. ELECTROOCULOGRAPHY

A definite potential difference is known to exist between the outer and inner sides of the retina or between the cornea and the sclera (Mowrer, Ruch, and Miller, 1936). Thus, during rotary movements of the eye in a horizontal plane, a change takes place in the potential difference between points of the skin lying to the right and left of the eye. When the eyes rotate in a vertical plane, these changes take place between points of the skin above and below the eye; they are produced in both cases by changes in the conditions of detection of the constant potential of the eye.

The changes in the potentials may be detected by a pair of electrodes fixed to corresponding points of the skin, and then amplified

and recorded. Since a linear relationship exists between the rotation
of the eye and the change in potential, the records obtained may easily
be used to determine the eye movements. It is essential in this method
that head movements do not influence the record of the eye movements
and that the record is made without contact with the eye. The main
disadvantage of the method is its low level of accuracy.

Miles (1939a, 1939b, 1940) investigated the action of various
conditions on the magnitude of the corneo-retinal potential difference
and showed that light adaptation causes an increase, dark adaptation
a decrease, in the potential difference. The potential changes recorded
were usually less than 1 millivolt.

Schott (1922), Meyers (1929), and Jacobson (1930a, 1930b) were
among the first investigators to use electrooculography to study the eye
movements. Later this method was widely adopted; it has been used
by Carmichael and Dearborn (1948), Monnier and Hufschmidt (1950),
Hodgson and Lord (1954), and others. In the Soviet Union, electrooculography was first used on a wide scale by L.T. Zagorul'ko, V.D.
Glezer, B. Kh. Gurevich, and L.I. Leushina at the I.P. Pavlov Institute
of Physiology in Leningrad.

The best of the electrooculographic methods suggested during recent
years would seem to be that described by Ford, White, and Lichtenstein (1959). By means of this method the horizontal and vertical
movements of the eye can be recorded simultaneously.

At the present time electrooculography is used with fair success by
many workers when highly accurate records of the eye movements are
not required (where the errors in the records may exceed 1°).

11. SOME PHOTOELECTRIC METHODS FOR RECORDING
EYE MOVEMENTS

Recently several authors have developed methods conventionally
known as photoelectric for recording eye movements.

One of the first methods of this type was devised by Dohlman
(1935). The scheme of this method was as follows. A source of light
and a photoelectric cell were affixed to the subject's head. Next, after
fixation of the lids, a rubber cup was affixed to the subject's anesthetized eye. The experimenter applied gentle pressure when placing the
cup on the eye, so that it easily remained in place by suction. A screen
was attached to the rubber cup, and this partly obstructed a beam of
light falling on the photoelectric cell.

The edge of the screen was situated so that the light was modulated
by the horizontal movements of the eyes. The amplified photoelectric

current was recorded, and the eye movements judged from its fluctuations.

Drischel and Lange (Drischel and Lange, 1956; Drischel, 1958) used the following method. A narrow band of infrared light was projected on the subject's eyes. The spot of light on the eye was 4 mm long and 1 mm wide. The light was directed towards the temporal side of the eye so that one half of the band was on the sclera and the other half on the iris. The iris absorbs light better than the sclera. Movement of the eyes caused modulation of the reflected light which fell on a photoelectric cell. The quantity of reflected light was directly related to the position of the eye. The current from the photoelectric cell was fed into an amplifier and then into an oscilloscope, from which photographic records were made.

Cornsweet (1958) developed the following method for investigating small movements of the eyes during fixation. After clamping the subject's head, a narrow beam of light was transmitted through the pupil onto the blind spot of the eye. The spot of light on the blind spot was shaped like a small rectangle. During movement of the eye, this spot intersected the large blood vessels, causing modulation of the reflected light. The reflected light was transmitted to a photomultiplier and oscilloscope, from which photographic records were made.

Smith and Warter (1959, 1960) suggested a simple variant of these methods. After the position of the subject's head had been fixed, an image of a small area of the eye was projected by an optical system on a horizontal slit. The center of this area corresponded to the boundary between the cornea and sclera at the point where the tangent to the boundary is vertical in position. In this case the image of the corneal border was perpendicular to the slit. The photocathode of a photomultiplier tube was placed behind the slit. Rotation of the eye around the vertical axis modulated the light falling on the photosensitive element of the tube. The recorded changes in the photoelectric current corresponded directly to the eye movements. Smith and Warter also described a moving object whose speed, brightness, and other characteristics may be modified at will. This system was connected with the system for recording eye movements so that the eye movements and the movements of the object were recorded simultaneously.

Gaarder (1960) used a method with a contact lens to which a plane mirror was fixed. A beam of light reflected from the mirror was transmitted to a photoelectric cell. By this method, both horizontal and vertical movements of the eyes could be recorded.

Shackel (1960) described a method which could be used to study the movements, not only of the eyes, but also of the head. A television camera, affixed to the subject's head recorded the field visible to the eye. The apparatus recording the eye movements transmitted to the same screen a small spot of white light corresponding, with a certain degree of accuracy, to the point of fixation at each particular moment.

Vladimirov and Khomskaya (1961) described a photoelectric method of recording eye movements giving a direct ink tracing. Via an optical system, the image of the subject's eye was projected on a piece of ground glass divided by a vertical screen into two equal parts. Behind each half of the ground glass was a photoresistor, the photosensitive layer of which was firmly in contact with the glass. Movement of the eye in the horizontal plane caused a displacement of its image on the ground glass and a change in the intensity of illumination of the photoresistors. The photoresistors were included in a circuit in which a change in the output voltage was directly proportional to the eye movement. This change was fed into the input of an amplifier or a loop. The horizontal movements of the eyes could be recorded with an accuracy of 1-2° by this method. As these authors state, their method is only suitable for recording the large movements of the eye.

Photoelectric methods can be used to study eye movements if an error of 1-2° is acceptable in the work. In nearly all these methods an increase in accuracy would require better fixation of the subject's head. Several of the photoelectric methods enable the eye movements to be studied without contact with the eye; this is their main advantage.

12. CREATION OF A STABILIZED RETINAL IMAGE WITH A CONTACT LENS

Ditchburn and Ginsborg (1952), and Riggs, Ratliff, Cornsweet, and Cornsweet (1953) describe a method designed to produce a stabilized image on the retina.

A rod is firmly fixed to a contact lens; at the end of the rod is a plane mirror. The rod is displaced relative to the axis of the lens so that the central part of the lens covering the cornea is left free and the blinking movement of the eye hardly impeded during the experiment. The axis of the rod, normal to the mirror, and axis of the lens are all parallel. After the lens has been fixed to the eye, a narrow beam of light is thrown from a projector on to the mirror. The beam reflected from the mirror enters the optical system and passes from it to a screen situated in front of the subject's eyes. The test field visible to the subject on the screen is circular and consists of two fields divided by a vertical boundary. The diameter of the test field is 2°. When the incident and reflected beams of light and the normal to the mirror remain in the same plane during eye movements, the angle of rotation of the reflected light is twice the angle of rotation of the eye. The optical system developed by these authors reduces the regular displacement of the image on the screen, making it equal in the horizontal direction to the rotation of the eye. The image of the vertical boundary between the two fields on the screen must remain stationary relative to the retina. Clowes and Ditchburn (1959) have improved this method so that it is possible to compensate not only the horizontal, but also the vertical component of the eye movements. These authors affixed a short-focus lens together with the test object to the contact lens. The short-focus lens was designed to produce a stationary and sharply defined image of the object on the retina.

The main disadvantage of methods creating a stationary retinal image by means of contact lenses is that during the experiment the vertical border on the test field disappears only for short intervals of time (several seconds). It then reappears for a few seconds and disappears again, and so on. The appearance of the boundary on the test field is perhaps due to insufficiently firm contact between the contact lens and the eye. Evidently, at times when the eye makes sudden rotations, the contact lens moves slightly and this leads to the appearance of the border.

13. SUCTION DEVICES (CAPS)

In this and the following sections of this chapter a description is given of the method used by the author of this book. The assembly of the appropriate instruments and accessories is described in one section.

The most important element of the apparatus used in this method is the special suction device, hereinafter referred to as a "cap." Depending on the object of the experiment, caps of different construction are made. Each cap is fixed during the experiment to the anesthetized surface of the subject's eye, causing no painful sensations or undesirable aftereffects. The method by which the cap is affixed to the eye is obvious from the description, suction device. The author claims that the cap ensures firm contact between the miniature apparatus used and the eye. In all experiments, the eyelids are secured to exclude blinking movements, which could displace the cap or detach it from the eye. No experiment should exceed a few minutes in duration.

When making the caps, several variations in shape and size are permissible. In most cases, therefore, illustrations of the caps are given not as scale drawings, but as schemes with explanations and

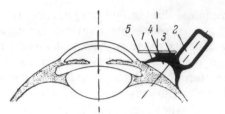

Fig. 13. The P_1 suction device or "cap."

indications of the more important measurements in the text. Each illustration of a cap must be regarded as a horizontal section passing through the optical axis of the right eye.

The construction of the caps is described with all necessary details to enable them to be made in any workshop. If the reader does not intend to make the cap and can readily grasp the idea of each construction with the description of its details, he may ignore this description. However, in order to understand the material in the following chapters, it is essential to have a general idea of the construction of each cap.

The cap shown schematically in Fig. 13 can be used to record eye movements. To simplify the descriptions, all caps of this type will be referred to in the future as type P_1. Any other type of cap will be denoted by the same letter but with a different index.

The P_1 cap is made of rubber. It consists of a round suction part 1, resembling an inverted dish, and a hollow cylindrical side-piece 2, joined by a canal 3 to a recess 4. A small mirror 5 is secured to the frame of the cap and used for recording the eye movements by reflecting a convergent beam of light. By means of the hollow side-piece, a reduced pressure is created inside the cap, and this facilitates its attachment to the sclera of the eye. After the cap has been fixed to the temporal part of the sclera, the surface of the mirror is approximately normal to the optical axis of the eye, and the hollow side-piece does not interfere with the incident and reflected beams of light during the experiment. The position of the cap can be seen from Fig. 13. The diameter of the suction part of large caps of type P_1 is 6-7 mm, that of small models, 3-4 mm. The size of the cap is determined by the size of the mirror required in the experiment. A change in the size of the cap is accompanied by a proportional change in all its dimensions. The diameter of the circular mirrors on the large models does not exceed 7-8 mm—3-4 mm, on the small. The thickness of the smallest mirrors is 0.2 mm, and that of the largest 0.3-0.4 mm. For some experiments, a rectangular mirror (5×7 mm) is more convenient. The length of the hollow side-piece is approximately equal to the diameter of the suction part. The external diameter of the hollow side-piece is equal to half its length and its thickness is 0.6-0.7 mm. The weight of the large caps, together with the mirror, is 0.20-0.25 g, and the weight of the small models 0.02-0.03 g. For most purposes, it is convenient to use a cap having a suction part 6 mm in diameter and a mirror of the same size.

The type P_2 cap is shown schematically in Fig. 14; it differs from the P_1 type only in shape and size. The P_2 cap is used when the eye has to be completely closed and at the same time its movements have to be recorded. The P_2 cap consists of a suction part (the frame) 1, the hollow side-piece 2, joined by the canal 3 to the recess 4. A mirror 5 is attached to the frame of the cap, and its surface is normal to the axis of symmetry of the frame and the optical axis of the eye. The measurements of the suction part and the measurements of the recess 4 are such that the cap nowhere touches the cornea. The height of the cap without the mirror is about 5.5-6 mm, and its external diameter is 13 mm. The hollow side-piece is 7-8 mm long, its external diameter is 4-5 mm, and the thickness of its walls is 0.5-0.6 mm. The mirror is 7-8 mm in diameter and 0.3 mm thick. The edge of the frame of the cap touching the sclera is not more than 0.2-0.3 mm thick. The middle part of the frame is 1.5-2 mm thick. The weight of the cap together with the mirror is 0.5-0.6 g.

A second variant of type P_2 is the P_3 cap, illustrated in Fig. 15. The only difference between this type and type P_2 is that its frame is made not of rubber but of thin duralumin. The P_3 model is much lighter than the P_2 and causes less irritation to the conjunctive. The dimensions of the frame are given in Fig. 15; they are identical with the dimensions of caps of several different types of construction. The surface of contact of the cap with the eye is polished and corrugated. The corrugated surface prevents the cap from slipping over the eye. The weight of the P_3 model is 0.20-0.25 g.

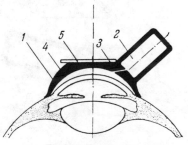

Fig. 14. The P_2 cap.

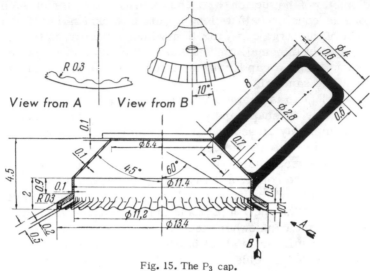

Fig. 15. The P_3 cap.

The P_4 cap is shown schematically in Fig. 16, and this model enables conditions of perception to be created in which the ordinary correlation between the eye movement and the displacement of the retinal image is disturbed. The duralumin frame of the P_4 cap has the same dimensions as the frame of the P_3 model. In the top part of the frame is a round aperture 1, with a diameter of 4 mm. A round glass plate 2 is fixed to the frame around its whole perimeter. To this glass plate is fixed a rectangular mirror 3, the plane of which makes an angle of 45° with the axis of symmetry of the frame of the apparatus. The dimensions of the mirror are 7 × 10 mm. When the cap is fixed to the eye, the subject can see an object only by means of the mirror.

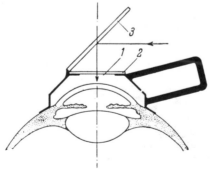

Fig. 16. The P_4 cap.

The hollow side-piece is so situated that the subject cannot see it in the mirror. All objects situated to the side appear to be displaced in the frontal plane. Rotation of the eye causes rotation of the mirror and, consequently, displacement of the retinal image. The relationship between the angle of rotation of the eye and the angle of displacement of the retinal image is very complex and differs sharply from what is found in normal conditions, i.e., when we look with the unaided eye. In other words, conditions are produced in which the subject clearly sees objects but cannot voluntarily choose points of fixation or use eye movements to obtain information concerning the spatial relationships between objects. The field of vision of an eye to which the P_4 apparatus is attached is approximately 50°. The weight of this cap is 0.30–0.35 g. If both large surfaces of the mirror of the P_4 apparatus are parallel and polished, by removing the reflecting layer a transparent window can be created in it. Through this window the subject can see objects in front of him (practically without distortion). When the P_4 apparatus with a window in the mirror is fixed to the eye, conditions are created in which the eye's field of vision is divided into two parts. In one part of this field, the ordinary relationship between the movement of the eye and displacement of the retinal image is disturbed, while in the other it is normal. To increase the sharpness of the border between the parts of the field, the size of the aperture 1 in the P_4 apparatus is reduced to 1.0–0.5 mm.

The P_5 cap, illustrated schematically in Fig. 17, is used to record the pulsations of the eye. The frame of the apparatus 2 and the hollow side-piece 14 are made of rubber. The hollow side-piece is joined by the opening 15 to the lower chamber 3 of the cap, in which is created the reduced pressure necessary for securing the apparatus to the eye.

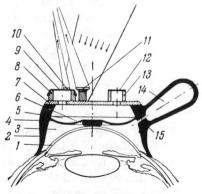

Fig. 17. The P_5 cap.

The lower chamber 3 of the cap is bounded below by the cornea of the eye 1, at the sides by the frame of the cap 2, and above by a thin rubber diaphragm 4 to which is secured a flat rubber button 6, lightly pressing on the cornea. The upper chamber 5 of the cap is bounded below by the rubber diaphragm 4, at the sides by the frame 2, and above by a rigid plate 7, fixed to the frame of the cap. The upper chamber is joined with the outside space through a special filter 12, fixed to a small cylinder 13. The filter transmits air slowly, so that the mean pressure in the chamber 5 is equal to atmospheric. The time taken for the pressure in the upper chamber to become equal is much greater than the blood pulsation period. Blood entering the eye causes pulsation of the intraocular pressure, and this in turn leads to deformation of the eye which is synchronized with the pulse. The deformation of the eye is transmitted to the elastic rubber diaphragm 4, movement of which causes a pulsation of pressure inside the upper chamber 5. The cylinder 8 is secured to the rigid plate 7. Over the cylinder 8 is gently stretched a very thin and elastic rubber membrane 9, several times thinner than the rubber diaphragm 4. The cylinder 8 is joined by an aperture with the upper chamber of the cap, so that pulsation of pressure inside the upper chamber is transmitted to the membrane 9 and deforms it synchronously with the pulsation of intraocular pressure. A small mirror 10 is fixed to the edge of the membrane 9. The mirror rotates during deformation of the membrane 9. Beside the mirror 10, secured to the membrane, is a mirror 11, rigidly fixed to the plate 7. A beam of light emerging from a slit aperture, reflected by both mirrors, and focused on the oscillographic paper of the photokymograph, records two lines. The beam of light reflected from the mirror 11, rigidly fixed to the cap, records the movements of the eye, while the beam of light reflected from the mirror 10, secured to the membrane, records the movements of the eye and the deformation of the cornea caused by the pulsation of intraocular pressure. In the course of the experiment the observer fixates on a certain point with his free eye. To ensure that the scale of the records is the same in all experiments, the distance between the observer's eye and the paper of the photokymograph is kept constant. In addition, before the cap is fixed in position, care must be taken that an approximately equal volume of air is withdrawn from the hollow side-piece. In external diameter, the frame of the P_5 cap is 13 mm. In its construction it resembles the frame of the P_2 model. When the pressure in the lower chamber 3 is equal to atmospheric and the apparatus rests with its edges on the sclera, the distance between the rubber diaphragm 4 and the cornea is 1.5-2.0 mm. The thickness of the diaphragm 4 is

0.2-0.3 mm. The diameter of the rubber button 6, fixed to the diaphragm, is 4 mm and its thickness 1 mm. The distance between the rubber diaphragm 4 and the rigid plate 7 is about 3 mm. The plate 7 is made of clear plastic 0.5 mm in thickness. The cylinders 8 and 13, of the same thickness, are made of clear plastic and glued to the plate. The internal diameter of cylinder 8 is 3 mm and of cylinder 13, 2 mm. The height of each cylinder and of the stand to which the mirror 11 is fixed is 3 mm. The diameters of the holes joining the spaces inside the cylinders 8 and 13 to the upper chamber 5 are each 1 mm. The thickness of the rubber membrane 9 stretched over cylinder 8 is about 0.03 mm. The mirrors 10 and 11 are square in shape, the first with a side of 1 mm and the second of 2 mm. The thickness of mirror 10 is 0.1 mm. Filter 12 is made of a single layer of ordinary filter paper and is glued to cylinder 13. The transmitting power of the filter is lowered by coating part of its surface with glue. The hollow side-piece 14 is 9 mm long; the external diameter of its lower part 5 mm and its upper part 6 mm, and the thickness of its walls is 0.7 mm. The weight of the P_5 cap is about 0.6-0.7 g. Assembly and preliminary adjustment of the cap are carried out on a rigid model of the eye, and final adjustments are made after experiments on the living eye and the necessary records have been obtained. During assembly it is important to select the correct tension of the diaphragm 4 and the membrane 9 and the correct transmitting capacity of the filter 12. It is, of course, easy to imagine a variant of the P_5 cap using a piezocrystal or any other suitable pickup. In this case, the recording of the pulsation could be made by means of an amplifier actuating a loop oscillograph.

The scheme of the P_6 cap, which creates a stationary retinal image for the whole field of vision of the eye, is shown in Fig. 18. The duralumin frame 1 and the hollow rubber side-piece 2 of the P_6 cap have the same dimensions as the frame and hollow side-piece of the P_3 model. The surface of contact between the frame and the eye is corrugated and polished. A thin duralumin cylinder 3, 0.1 mm thick, is glued firmly to the frame. The diameter of the cylinder and its height are about 5 mm. Inside the cylinder are mounted two duralumin diaphragms 4, in firm contact with it. Each diaphragm is 0.1 mm thick, and the diameter of the aperture is 1.5-2.5 mm. The diameter of the aperture in the upper part of the frame of the apparatus is 2.5-3 mm. The distance between the frame and the first diaphragm is 1 mm, and that between the frame and the second diaphragm 2 mm. A short-focus lens 5 is fixed to the second diaphragm and the cylinder. The focal length of the lens is 5-8 mm. Over the cylinder 3 is placed a device conventionally called an adaptor. The frame of the adaptor is

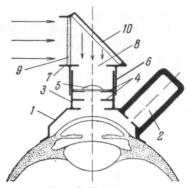

Fig. 18. The P_6 cap.

made of black paper. The lower part of the adaptor consists of the
paper cylinder 6, which is firmly held by friction on the duralumin
cylinder 3. A paper square 7 with a round hole 8 in the center is glued
to the cylinder 6. The side of the square 7 is a few millimeters longer
than the diameter of the paper cylinder 6, and the hole 8, in turn, is a
few millimeters smaller than this diameter, and is in fact 3.5 mm.
The hole in the square is situated at the focus of the lens. The test field
fits into the hole. A square frosted glass (side 6 mm long), about
0.2 mm thick, is fixed parallel to one side of the square 7 and perpendicular to its plane. The mirror 10, 6 mm wide (the same size as the
frosted glass), 9 mm high, and 0.1–0.2 mm thick, is fixed at an angle
of 45° to the paper square and the frosted glass. Triangular pieces of
black paper are fixed to the edges of the frosted glass and the mirror
so that the inside of the adaptor receives light only through the frosted
glass. All the slits in the adaptor are carefully glued together, and the
device is painted black.

During the experiment the adaptor occupies the position shown in
Fig. 18. Experiments with the P_6 cap are usually carried out in a dark
room. A narrow beam of light, shown by arrows in Fig. 18, falls only
on the adaptor of the cap and illuminates the frosted glass. The sclera
of the eye is practically in total darkness, and, consequently, light
enters the eye only through the cap, a very important factor in many
experiments with an image stationary relative to the retina.

The short-focus lens gives a magnified image of the test field which
the eye sees against the background of the frosted glass reflected in the
mirror. Adjustment of the sharpness of the image is done by moving
the adaptor along the duralumin cylinder 3. It is clear from Fig. 18
that the lens of the apparatus is housed inside the cylinder a short
distance from the cornea and separated from it by the diaphragm.

This type of construction was determined by the need for protecting the lens against clouding, which would have interfered with the conduct of the experiment. Since the short-focus lens gives high magnification, the visible diameter of the test field may be made greater than 50°. As mentioned above, the test field and the projection system of the P_6 apparatus are firmly fixed to its frame. The frame of the cap, in turn, is firmly fixed to the eye and, consequently, even during movement of the eyes the retinal image of the test field is always stationary relative to the retina. The weight of the P_6 cap without the adaptor is 0.15-0.20 g.

The P_7 cap, by means of which two superposed retinal images may be obtained on the retina, is illustrated schematically in Fig. 19. One of the two images is stationary relative to the retina while the other is movable.

The duralumin frame 1 of the P_7 model and the hollow rubber bulb 2 are the same size as the frame and the hollow bulb of the P_3 apparatus. The contact surface between the frame and the eye is corrugated and polished. To the whole perimeter of the frame is fixed a duralumin cylinder 3, with an external diameter of 5 mm, a height of 2 mm, and walls 0.1 mm thick. Inside the cylinder is fixed a duralumin diaphragm 4. The thickness of the diaphragm is 0.1 mm and the diameter of the aperture 3.5 mm. The distance between diaphragm 4 and the frame is 1 mm. The diameter of the aperture 5 in the upper part of the frame is 3 mm. A round transparent glass 6 with the lens 7 is fixed to the cylinder 3 around its entire perimeter. The glass is 6 mm in diameter and 0.15-0.20 mm thick. The diameter of the lens is 2-3 mm and its focal length 5-8 mm. The cylinder 3 is so made that it removes the glass with the lens a short distance from the eye and thus prevents it from becoming steamed up. A round wooden rod 8 is fixed to the frame of the cap and the cylinder. In turn, the test

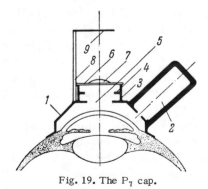

Fig. 19. The P_7 cap.

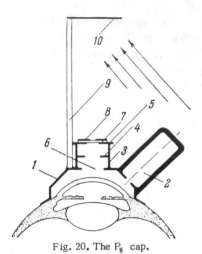

Fig. 20. The P_8 cap.

field 9 is fixed to the rod and is stationary relative to the rod and to the frame of the cap. The height of the rod is determined by the focal length of the lens and is so designed that a sharp image of the test field 9 may be obtained on the retina. It is clear from Fig. 19 that lens 7 covers only the central part of the glass 6, leaving the peripheral part open. When the cap is fixed to the eye, the peripheral part of the glass (the circular diaphragm) enables the subject to see clearly and to examine the surrounding object freely. The color contrast of the visible objects is slightly below normal due to the scattered light (the out-of-focus image of surrounding objects) falling on the retina through the lens. The lens gives a sharp retinal image of the test field fixed to the rod, and since it is firmly connected to the cap, this image is strictly stationary relative to the retina. As a result, two images, superposed on each other, are formed on the retina. One is movable relative to the retina (movable because of the eye movements) while the other is strictly stationary and unchanged in color (provided that the illumination of test field 9 is unchanged). By changing the area of the circular diaphragm and the diameter of the lens, the brightness of the stationary and moving retinal images may be varied within certain limits.

The scheme of the P_8 cap, by means of which images remain stationary relative to the retina for any part of the field of vision of the eye, is illustrated in Fig. 20.

The duralumin frame 1 of the P_8 model and the hollow rubber bulb 2 are the same size as the frame and the bulb of the P_3 cap. The surface of contact between the frame and the eye is corrugated and polished. Around the whole perimeter of the frame is fixed the duralumin

cylinder 3.   The external diameter of the cylinder is 4.5 mm, its
height 3 mm, and the thickness of its wall 0.1 mm. Inside the cylinder
is fixed the duralumin diaphragm 4.   The diaphragm 5 is 0.1 mm
thick, and its aperture is 2 mm in diameter. The cylinder is closed
on top by a second diaphragm 5, which is fixed to the cylinder around
its whole perimeter.   Diaphragm 5 is 0.1 mm thick, its external
diameter is 5 mm, and the diameter of the aperture is 1.5 mm. The
diameter of the aperture 6 in the upper part of the frame of the apparatus is 2.5 mm.   The distance between the diaphragm 4, situated
inside the cylinder, and the frame of the cap is 1.5 mm. A round
transparent glass 7 is glued all around the perimeter of the second
diaphragm 5.   This glass is 0.1-0.2 mm thick and 4 mm in diameter.
Interchangeable diaphragms 8, made of thin black paper or foil, are
glued to the glass.   Depending on the object of the experiment, the
apertures of the interchangeable diaphragms vary from 0.2 to 1.5 mm.
A rod 9 (a thin steel wire), to which is fixed the screen 10—the test field
stationary relative to the frame of the apparatus—is fixed to the frame
of the cap and to the cylinder.   The height of the rod (usually about
20-25 mm) is determined by the purpose of the experiment. Cylinder
3 and the first two diaphragms 4 and 5 are designed so as to keep
the glass from steaming up.

When the cap is fixed to the eye, the screen becomes stationary
relative to the retina. The small size of the aperture of diaphragm 8,
fixed to the glass, increases the depth of focus to such a degree that,
besides objects at a distance from the eye, the screen 10 can also be
clearly seen. The sharpness of the image of the screen depends on
the size of the aperture in the diaphragm. The smaller the aperture
in the diaphragm, the sharper the image of the screen. However,
reducing the size of the diaphragm aperture also diminishes the brightness of the visual image.   For this reason, in each experiment a
diaphragm is chosen which is satisfactory for the experimenter as
regards both the sharpness of the screen's image and the brightness
of objects visible to the eye.   Some increase in the sharpness of
definition of the image of the screen can be obtained by lengthening
the rod, i.e., by moving the screen further from the eye, but with this
manoeuvre, the rigidity of the connection between the screen and the
frame of the apparatus and between the frame of the cap and the eye
is rapidly lost. By giving the screen different shapes and positions
in space, it is comparatively easy to produce a stationary retinal image
of a given shape and color in any part of the retina. To increase the
brightness of the screen, a beam of light is thrown upon it, as shown
by the arrows in Fig. 20. If a filter instead of a screen is affixed to

the rod, conditions of perception are produced in which a definite part of the retina is shielded by the filter. Because of the small mirror fixed to the cylinder of the P_8 cap, eye movements can be recorded under conditions in which a given part of the retina is shielded by the screen, i.e., is in fact prevented from receiving any visual stimulation.

Depending on the purpose of the investigation, the experimenter may need to modify not only the construction of the caps, but also the construction of the adaptors. The descriptions in the second chapter of certain experiments include a detailed account of several adaptors used with the P_6 apparatus.

14. APPARATUS USED IN WORK WITH CAPS

A photograph of the apparatus usually used in recording eye movements is given in Fig. 21. The apparatus consists of a stand (or frame), a chin rest, two light sources, and a control panel. The frame consists basically of a large, massive stand.

Two metal uprights and the control panel, on which sockets and switches are mounted, are firmly fixed to this stand. On the movable part of the large stand is mounted a metal post ending in a chin rest. The chin rest can be moved vertically; horizontally, it can turn about the axis of the post, and after the desired position has been obtained, it can be firmly fixed. In addition, the parameters of the chin rest itself may be varied by the experimenter, depending on the size of the subject's head. By use of this type of chin rest, the subject's head can be securely fixed during the experiments. On each metal post is a massive connecting rod, and at the end of this rod a universal stand. The light source is fixed on ball bearings to each stand. By means of this system the experimenter can quickly (and this is very important) direct a beam of light reflected from the mirror of the cap to the aperture of a kymograph or to a cassette. The switchboard control panel permits any apparatus to be switched on and off in the course of the experiment without interrupting the observation.

Depending on which cap is used for the experiment and the particular purpose of the investigation, the experimenter will need to use different light sources and accessories. For example, when recording eye movements on still photosensitive paper or film, a light source is used which throws a spot of light not more than 1 mm in diameter onto the photosensitive material. In this case the objective gives an image of the small aperture of the diaphragm against the background of the incandescent filament. Usually a series of diaphragms with

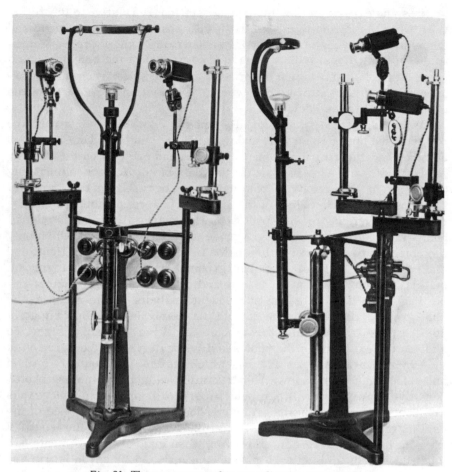

Fig. 21. The apparatus used in recording eye movements.

apertures between 10 and 70 μ in diameter is used in an investigation. If the eye movements are recorded on a photokymograph, a slit takes the place of the diaphragm in the light source; the slits in a suitable series vary from 10 to 70 μ in width.

To illuminate the frosted glass of the P_6 apparatus or the screen in the P_8 apparatus, a light source is used which has an optical system allowing a beam of light about 10–15 mm in diameter to be obtained at any point in space, illuminating a small area of surface uniformly. Uniformity of illumination is essential to ensure that during eye movements, i.e., during movements of the frosted glass or the screen, their brightness does not change within the beam of light.

In some experiments with an image stationary relative to the retina (i.e., when the P_6 and P_8 models are used), adaptors with polarized and other different types of filters are attached to the light sources. Sometimes special discs and vanes are used to change the brightness and color of the light falling on the frosted glass or the screen in accordance with a given pattern. However, no explanation is required of the construction of these devices.

When using the P_6, P_7, and P_8 types of cap, the experiments are best carried out in conditions under which the subject's face is turned upward, and the fixation point for the second eye lies on the ceiling. An armchair with a low back, with a controllable device for maintaining the head in the required position, may be used for this purpose.

Depending on the object of the experiment, eye movements may be recorded on moving or still photosensitive material. Records on still photographic paper or film are made in a dark room, in which only the object of perception is illuminated by a directed beam of light, and placed against a black matt background. Usually the photographic material is enclosed in a cassette and opened only during actual recording. To facilitate the subsequent analysis of the records, the photographic paper or film should be fairly large, approximately 30×40 cm. The cassettes should be of corresponding size. To shorten the exposure of the photosensitive material and the duration of the experiment, cassettes are used which are easily and quickly opened and closed in a dark room. When records are made on moving photosensitive material (oscillographic paper), ordinary photokymographs are used. However, in the ordinary photokymograph the speed of the oscillographic paper does not exceed 20-30 cm/sec and the length of the slit is only 12-15 cm. However, when many eye movements are studied, speeds closer to 5 m/sec and slits 25-30 cm in length are necessary. These technical conditions are satisfied by a primitive and somewhat modified model of a photokymograph, the making of which presents no special difficulty and requires no detailed description. Such a photokymograph is based on a large drum, to which wide oscillographic paper is fixed in darkness. The diameter of the drum is 50-60 cm, and its height is determined by the width of the oscillographic paper, which should be at least 25-30 cm wide. The axle of the drum is connected to an electric motor through a gearbox or reducing chain. The whole system is covered with a lightproof plywood case with a slit surrounded by visors preventing scattered light from falling on the drum. The gearbox allows the speed of rotation of the drum to be changed. The linear velocities of the oscillographic paper may be varied in this manner from several centimeters to several meters per second. Repeated turns of the drum cause the records to be superposed on each other. Of course, the experiment must be stopped before the whole picture becomes too confused and too complicated for analysis. The higher the speed, the shorter the experiment must be. When the speed of the oscillographic paper is several meters per second, in many cases recording should not continue longer than 10-20 sec.

When it is necessary to affix apparatus essential for or facilitating an experiment to the subject's face, he wears a Plexiglas mask, as shown in Fig. 22. The mask fits the face and head snugly and stays in position satisfactorily. A number of holes with a screw thread are made in the Plexiglas to which the experimenter may attach the required accessories.

Besides those mentioned above, apparatuses familiar in laboratory practice may also be used in work with caps.

15. TECHNIQUE OF EXPERIMENTS WITH CAPS

The cap cannot remain on the subject's eye more than a few minutes. As soon as the cap has been fixed to the eye, the work to be done falls into two parts—adjustment of the apparatus, and the experiment itself. In many cases the adjustment of the apparatus is itself complicated and takes much time.

Very careful preparation for each experiment can minimize this time. Preparation for working with the caps begins with the choice of subject. The subject should have large eyes, a long palpebral fissure and his conjunctiva should be healthy and not irritated by amethocaine.

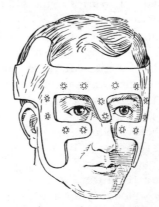

Fig. 22. Plexiglas mask for attachment of accessories used in experiments with caps.

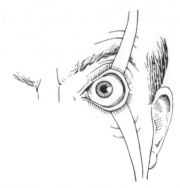

Fig. 23. Position of lids held by strips of adhesive plaster in work with the P_1 cap.

The experimenter should first make a detailed plan of the experiment, prepare every piece of equipment required, and give the subject his instructions. The subject sits with his chin on the chin rest or in the special armchair. After preliminary adjustment of the whole apparatus, it is tested to make sure that it is ready. This is particularly important when eye movements are recorded on still photographic paper or film. Correct positioning of the visual test object and the cassette relative to the subject simplifies the experiment and reduces distortion.

The experimenter then cuts strips of adhesive plaster for holding back the eyelids. Each strip is 12-15 mm wide and about 10 cm long. Usually two strips are sufficient for the lids of one eye. The prepared strips of adhesive plaster are placed on a clean sheet of paper. The whole sheet of paper with the strips is placed on a surface kept heated to a temperature of 60-80°C, where it stays until required. Heating the adhesive plaster causes it to stick to the skin more firmly and hold the eyelids more securely.

Next, the experimenter wipes the subject's eyelids, forehead, and cheeks with cotton wool lightly soaked in alcohol, making the skin dry and clean. He then instils two or three drops of a 1% solution of amethocaine into the conjunctival sac, wipes away the tears with dry cotton wool, and after 1-2 minutes proceeds to tape back the eyelids. This is done as follows. The subject is asked to close his eyes and one end of a strip of adhesive plaster is pressed against the upper lid so that it touches the eyelashes. By pressing the skin of the eyelids covered with adhesive plaster with two fingers, the lid is retracted together with the plaster from the eye until a vertical fold is formed between the fingers. By squeezing the fold, a firm connection between the adhesive plaster and skin is obtained. By pulling on the other end of the strip of adhesive plaster, the lid may be raised to the required position and held there by sticking the strip to the forehead. The lower lid is taped in precisely the same way, except that the strip of adhesive plaster is stuck to the cheek. If the subject wears the mask (Fig. 22), the strips of adhesive plaster may be stuck to it. The position of the lids for working with the P_1 type of cap is illustrated in Fig. 23, and the position of the lids for working with all other types of cap in Fig. 24. In the first case, as is clear from Fig. 23, the lids are retracted mainly towards the temporal part of the eye. In the second case, the adhesive plaster is stuck to the central part of each eyelid and the lids are retracted almost symmetrically relative to the optical axis.

After the lids have been fixed, the subject places his head on the chin rest in the required position, and the experimenter applies the cap to the eye.

To apply the cap, the experimenter holds it by the bulb with his two fingers, squeezes the air from it, places it in the required position, gently pressing the suction part to the eye, and releases the bulb. The re-expanding bulb lowers the pressure inside the cap, and the external pressure presses it firmly against the sclera.

Later the experimenter places the light sources in the correct position, makes sure that all the apparatus is in working order, and begins the experiment. The different experiments differ considerably in their complexity, although all demand skill and precision from the experimenter in his work. Recording eye movements on still photographic paper or film is complicated. Let us assume that the cap is fixed to the eye. The cassette is still closed but ready to record. The room is dark. The visual test object, placed against a matt black background, is illuminated by a directed beam of light but covered by paper so that the subject cannot see it before recording begins. Then the

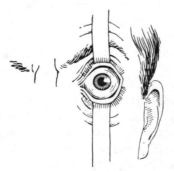

Fig. 24. Position of lids held by strips of adhesive plaster in work with all caps except type P_1.

command is given, and the subject fixates on the center of the visual test object. The experimenter moves the light source, and directs the beam of light reflected from the mirror of the cap to the center of the cassette. Next, the subject moves his glance several times around the borders of the object. The experimenter, watching the movements of the light spot over the cassette, moves the cassette (and sometimes both the cassette and the light source) to a point in space at which the whole record can be accommodated on the photosensitive material, and distortions in the record are minimal. The subject then again fixates on the center of the test object. The experimenter obtains a sharp image of the light spot on the cassette. Before recording begins, the subject fixates on a point situated at a distance from the the test object so that the light spot does not move off the cassette. The experimenter uncovers the cassette and the test object, switches on the second counter, and tells the subject to look at the test object. After a certain period of time, the experimenter switches off the light and the record comes to an end. The cassette is then closed, the light is switched on, the subject's face is illuminated, and the cap and the strips of adhesive plaster are removed. The cassette is then taken to the photographic laboratory for processing and analysis.

The cap is removed from the eye as follows: the subject is asked to fixate on a certain point so as to prevent eye movement, the hollow bulb is compressed with two fingers, expelling all the air from it, and the cap can then be removed from the eye.

When the cap is attached to the eye, the subject must restrict his eye movements to avoid knocking the cap against the lids. Usually, at the beginning of the experiment, the experimenter indicates the limits of the field beyond which the subject must not choose points of fixation. If it comes into contact with the lids, the cap may be detached from the eye or may be displaced so that its suction part is on the cornea, and, worst of all, it may injure the eye. This must always be borne in mind by both experimenter and subject.

As a rule the duration of experiments with the cap should not exceed 5 min, and only in rare cases as long as 10-12 min. When working with the P_1 type of cap, observations must be made constantly on the state of the cornea, for in some subjects it begins to dry after only 3 min. Drying of the cornea, especially its central part, is accompanied by a sharp fall in the resolving power of the eye and is always regarded by the subject with some alarm. In such cases, the experiment must be stopped. The cornea usually resumes its previous form after a few minutes. The P_1 cap itself cannot injure the eyes. The worst it can do is to rupture a superficial blood vessel in the conjunctiva. This suggests that the particular subject is not suitable. The

P_1 cap always causes a slight fall of intraocular pressure, but this is restored after 1 or a few hours, and the subject feels no sensations associated with the change of pressure. In people with a normal intra-ocular pressure, the pressure falls approximately 1-2 mm Hg; in patients with glaucoma, the intraocular pressure may fall by several millimeters.

All types of cap except P_1 protect the cornea against drying but compress the blood vessels in the conjunctiva around the whole perim-eter of the cornea. For this reason experiments with the large caps likewise should not exceed the time mentioned above. Usually, even if the subject feels well, experiments should not be performed every day, but every other day, and not more than one or two experiments should be carried out with each eye. If all the rules are observed and if due attention is paid to the subject, work with the caps is quite free from risk, and the subject will feel no particularly unpleasant sen-sations after several experiments. The author has used a number of subjects now for several years. No adverse results caused by work with the caps have been observed.

The photographic material is processed by the usual methods available in any photographic laboratory. In particular, rephotography is sometimes used to reduce distortions, and retouching, decolorizing, and so on may be required to increase contrast.

16. COURSE OF THE RAYS IN RECORDING EYE MOVEMENTS BY A REFLECTED BEAM OF LIGHT

We will now examine in detail the main distortions and errors which may be encountered when eye movements are recorded by means of a mirror. Let us assume that:

1. The center of rotation of the eye is stationary, as is the ob-server's head.

2. The reflecting surface of the plane mirror lies in the center of rotation of the eye and is firmly connected to it.

3. The surface of the mirror is always normal to the optical axis of the eye.

4. The light source is stationary. Axial rays from the light source pass through the center of rotation of the eye.

5. A spherical photosensitive surface is made, the center of which coincides with the center of rotation of the eye.

Let us now imagine a series of planes passing through the axis of the objective of the light source and the rotation center of the eye. For all eye movements in which a line that is normal to the rotating mirror

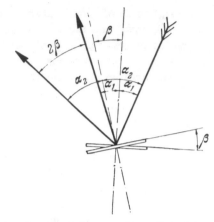

Fig. 25. Scheme showing the path of the rays when reflected from a plane rotating mirror.

(and the optical axis) moves in one of the planes mentioned above, we obtain a record on the photosensitive surface of the sphere which differs from the ideal only in the fact that each angle of rotation of the optical axis is doubled by the reflected light.

In fact, let us assume that at a certain moment of time the angle between the incident beam of light and the line normal to the mirror is a_1 (Fig. 25); the incident beam of light and the line normal to the mirror are situated in the plane of the drawing. Since the angle of incidence is equal to the angle of reflection, consequently the angle between the incident and reflected beam of light will be $2a_1$. Let us assume further that at some later moment the mirror is turned through an angle β or, what amounts to the same thing, a line normal to its surface is turned through an angle β. The angle between the incident beam of light and the line normal to the mirror will then be $a_1 + \beta = a_2$, while the angle between the incident beam of light and the reflected beam will now be $2a_2 = 2a_1 + 2\beta$. Hence it follows that when the mirror is turned through an angle β, the reflected beam of light is turned through an angle $(2a_1 + 2\beta) - 2a_1 = 2\beta$.

Some distortion of the record is produced by the fact that the mirror is not in the rotation center of the eye, but on its surface. Let us consider two cases: (a) the line normal to the mirror coincides with the optical axis when we use the P_2 or P_3 type of cap (Fig. 26); and (b) the line normal to the mirror is parallel to the optical axis, but at a certain distance from it when the P_1 cap is used (Fig. 27).

Let us assume that the axis of rotation of the eye is perpendicular to the plane of the drawing, and that the visual axis, which is normal to the mirror, and the axis of the light source are also in this plane. Let us assume that a collimated beam of light emerges from the stationary light source, and that its width is equal to the diameter of the eye, so that in both cases the rotation center of the reflected beam of light will be shifted in space as indicated in Figs. 26 and 27. The rotation center of the optical axis is stationary; the reflected beam of light, turned through an angle twice as great as the angle of rotation of the eye, receives an additional movement due to displacement of the mirror (see Fig. 26). In the initial position, when $a = 0$, the beam of light reflected from the mirror situated in the center of rotation is combined with the beam of light reflected from the mirror situated on the surface of the eye. If the eye is rotated, for example, through an angle of a_1 or a_2, the reflected beams are rotated, respectively, through angles of $2a_1$ and $2a_2$, and they are also displaced through a distance of A_1 and A_2.

A similar picture may be observed in Fig. 27. In the initial position, when $a = 0$, the beam of light reflected from the mirror situated at the center of rotation is displaced relative to the beam of light reflected from a mirror situated on the eye surface by the distance A_0. When the eye is rotated, for example through an angle of a_1 and a_2, the reflected beams are rotated correspondingly through angles of $2a_1$ and $2a_2$ and, in addition, they may be superposed (at a_1) or displaced (at a_2, by a distance A_2). However, collimated beams of light are not

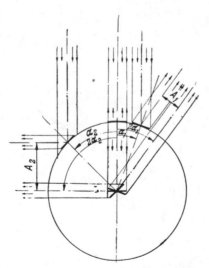

Fig. 26. Scheme showing the path of the rays when reflected from a plane mirror rotating and undergoing displacement in space, illuminated by a collimated beam of light. The case when the P_2 or P_3 type of cap is used.

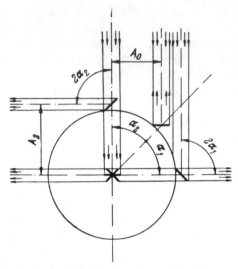

Fig. 27. Scheme showing the path of the rays when reflected from a plane mirror rotating and undergoing displacement in space, illuminated by a collimated beam of light. The case when the P_1 cap is used.

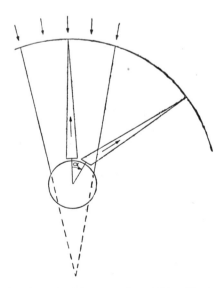

Fig. 28. Scheme showing the path of the rays when reflected from a plane mirror, rotating and undergoing displacement in space, illuminated by a convergent beam of light.

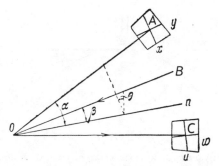

Fig. 29. Explanatory scheme for considering the transformation of coordinates when recording
by a beam of light reflected from a mirror.

used in the experiments. By means of the ordinary objective, the
image of a very small aperture of the diaphragm or narrow slit is
projected on the screen, and the path of the rays in these conditions
will be as shown in Fig. 28.

With small angles of rotation of the eye (less than 10°) and a large
enough radius of the spherical surface on which the record is made,
the distortions obtained as a result of displacement of the mirror in
space and defocusing are negligibly small by comparison with the
displacements of the image of the diaphragm aperture arising on
account of rotation of the mirror, i.e., on account of eye movement.

To represent the way in which movements of the projection of the
optical axis of the eye are transformed at the plane of the object into
movements of the ray of light reflected from the mirror on to photosensitive paper, let us examine Fig. 29.

Let us assume that OA is the axis of vision, On the normal to the
mirror, OB the direction of a beam of light falling on the mirror, OC
the direction of the reflected beam of light, a the angle between the
axis of vision and the line normal to the mirror, β the angle between
the axis of the incident beam of light and the normal to the mirror,
and θ the angle between two planes, one of which passes through the
axis of vision and the line normal to the mirror and the other through
the direction of the incident beam and the normal to the mirror.

Let x and y represent the coordinates of the object to be examined,
and u and w the coordinates of the ray of light reflected on to photosensitive paper, normal relative to the ray. The axes are chosen so
that Ax is the projection of the plane AOn on the plane of the object,
and the axis Cu is the projection of the plane nOC on the plane of the
image. By simple geometry we reach the following relationships
between the coordinates:

$$u = 2(x \cos\theta - y \cos a \sin\theta), \quad w = 2(x \cos\beta \sin\theta + y \cos a \cos\beta \cos\theta).$$

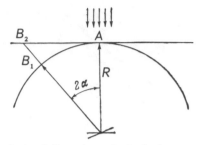

Fig. 30. Scheme for analysis of distortions obtained when recording eye movements on a plane rather than a spherical surface.

These equations are valid for small displacements x and y. With larger displacements the transformation becomes more complex (not affine, but projective).

The expressions for u and w show how distortions arise when eye movements are recorded by a beam of light reflected from a mirror at certain definite values of a, β, and θ. It is easy to see that the smaller the angles a and β the smaller the distortions obtained on recording. At the limit when $a = 0$, $\beta = 0$, we have $u = 2x$ and $w = 2y$. When $a = 0$ or $\beta = 0$, the angle θ is not determine. In this case we obtain formally the transformation of the rotation through an arbitrary angle. This corresponds to the fact that in such cases there is no determinacy in the choice of the x or u axes. By suitable choice, if $a = 0$ and $\beta = 0$, the equation may be represented in the form $u = 2x$ and $w = 2y$.

Usually, eye movements are not recorded on a spherical photo-sensitive surface, but on a plane surface (Fig. 30). Let the axis of rotation of the eye be perpendicular to the plane of the drawing and let the axis of vision, the normal to the mirror, and the axis of illumina-tion lie in this plane. Let the reflected ray be initially at the point A. When the mirror is rotated through an angle a, the reflected ray moves to point B_2. In this case, distortion of the recording is obtained because the path of the ray to the plane surface (AB_2) is longer than the path traversed by the ray to the sphere (AB_1). It follows from this drawing that with small angles the distortions indicated above are small and may be ignored. When the record is made on a plane surface, the distortions obtained may be calculated, and appropriate corrections may be made when the photographs are analyzed.

In this discussion of eye movements, the course of the rays, and the accuracy of the records, we have to some extent idealized the whole picture. We have not taken into consideration the fact that some move-ment of the head in reality always remains. During movement of the eye the center of its rotation is slightly displaced, i.e., displacement of the eye relative to the orbit takes place. In addition, the eye is displaced slightly in the orbit because of the pulsation of blood, which also gives rise to a slight pulsating deformation of the eye itself. In most cases, however, none of these factors have much effect on the records made by a reflected beam of light.

17. CONSTRUCTION OF CAPS

The rubber parts of the caps are turned on a lathe with the arbor turning at high speeds (5000-6000 rpm), from ordinary rubber (for example, rubber stoppers). The tools required include cutting tools, files, nail files, metal templates, emery paper, and so on. The initial stage of work on the lathe is done with the file, by means of which the correct diameter of the blank is obtained. The cutting tools, the nail files, and the metal template are used to give the part its rough finish. Later, each rubber part is polished with emery paper. The part itself is continually moistened with benzene during this process, making the rubber pliable for a short time but easily polished. In the last operation the revolving detail is cut away from the blank by a sharp scalpel. Since the rubber details are turned at high speeds, and the tool is as a rule unsupported except by the experimenter's hands, the appropriate safety regulations must be strictly observed.

The holes in the rubber part of the caps are made either with a very small drill (a metal tube with one sharpened end) or with a thread. A thread is passed through with a fine needle, pulled tight, and fixed in a vertical position; the thread is soaked in benzene, and the rubber part is moved along it so that the direction of the hole and the direction of the thread coincide. After the rubber has been moved up and down the thread soaked in benzene several times, a hole is made which is approximately equal to the thread in diameter.

The mirrors fixed to the caps must possess good optical properties. This applies primarily to the mirrors by means of which the drift and tremor of the eye are recorded. The mirrors must have no sharp edges or corners. Since the outer surface of the reflecting layer is used in the experiments, aluminum mirrors are more practical than silver-coated mirrors. The silver coating quickly darkens and loses the properties of a mirror surface.

The P_1 model is assembled from its finished part by means of universal glue (for example, No. 88 glue) on a rigid life-size model of the eye. Assembly on the model ensures that the mirror and the bulb of the apparatus are in the correct position. BF-2 glue is best for affixing the paper adaptors, and for bonding glass to metal, metal to metal, and glass to paper. No. 88 glue should be used for gluing rubber to itself, to glass, or to metal.

The duralumin frame of the models P_3-P_8 is turned on a small lathe on which work can be done under a binocular loupe. Ordinary small cutting tools are used. The cutting surfaces of these tools must be very sharp. The sharper the tools, the thinner the parts can be made.

It was pointed out earlier that the surface of contact between the metal cap and the sclera is corrugated and polished. This corrugation is produced on a lathe, during the first stage in manufacture of the frame, while the blank still possesses considerable mechanical strength. After the surface has been corrugated, the following operations are carried out without changing the position and angle of rotation of the support. Thirty-six marks are made on the cylindrical surface of the chuck so that the distance between two adjacent marks corresponds to a rotation of the arbor by 10°. A cutting tool shaped in such a way that a groove of the required shape and size is planed out when the support is brought up is fixed in the support. By using the grooves and turning the arbor each time through 10°, 36 grooves are made. In the next operation the grooves are polished, at first each one separately, and then all together, changing the direction of rotation of the arbor in turn. After the corrugated surface has been polished, the frame of the cap is then finished in the usual way.

It is sometimes difficult to obtain a short-focus lens of the required focal length. A method of making these lenses is given below. The wide end of a glass drop has an almost ideal spherical shape, and can therefore be used as the blank for making a lens. The work begins by producing glass drops of different diameters. These drops may easily be obtained from any glass blower's workshop. The order of the operations which should be followed when making the lenses is given in Fig. 31. First the glass drops are coated with a thin layer of casein glue, and this is allowed to dry. The glue protects the surface of the future lens from injury. A small metal washer is then made, the hole in which is slightly larger than the diameter of the drop, and its thickness is equal to the thickness of the future lens. A piece of glass is glued to one side of the hole in the washer. The glass drop is placed inside the washer as shown in the figure, and all the free space in the hole is filled with liquid Canada balsam. The solidified balsam holds the drop firmly inside the washer. Next, the part of the glass drop projecting from the hole in the washer is ground down with emery paper. Towards the end of this operation, emery paper of very fine grain is used to make the plane surface of the lens smoother. A thin

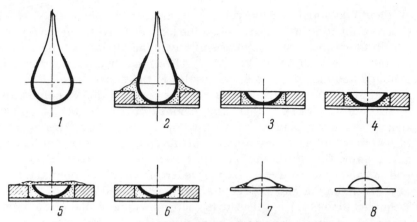

Fig. 31. Scheme to explain the processes of making short-focus lenses. Order of operations—
1) a glass drop is coated with glue to protect its spherical surface from injury; 2) the drop
is placed inside a washer and affixed to it with Canada balsam; 3) the part of the drop
projecting from the hole in the washer is ground down with emery paper; 4) part of the
Canada balsam is removed with the grains of glass; 5) the space inside the washer is again
completely filled with Canada balsam; 6) the plane surface of the lens is polished; 7) the
lens is carefully cleaned to remove Canada balsam and glue and then glued to a glass cover
slip with Canada balsam; 8) Canada balsam is removed from the exposed surfaces of the
cover slip and from the spherical surface of the lens; all surfaces are carefully rubbed
clean.

layer of Canada balsam is then removed with a piece of cotton wool
soaked in alcohol, in order to ensure that all grains of glass rubbed
off by the emery paper are removed. This is necessary to prevent
scratching of the lens surface during polishing by loose grains of glass.
The space around the lens is then filled again with a drop of liquid
Canada balsam. Excess balsam is removed with cotton wool soaked
in alcohol, and the plane surface of the lens is then polished.

A piece of clean cotton cloth is drawn over the glass, it is coated
with paste, and the lens is polished by moving the washer on the cloth.
If the experimenter does not possess the special paste, paste for strop-
ping razors may be used. After this polishing, the lens surface will
not be ideally flat, but it should have no scratch marks or pits. After
polishing, the Canada balsam is dissolved, and the lens is taken out of
the washer. The casein glue is removed from the lens surface with
hot water. The plane surface of the lens is carefully wiped dry and in
the next operation it is glued to a previously prepared round glass
cover slip with Canada balsam. Next, the excess Canada balsam is
removed from the exposed surfaces of the cover slip and from the
spherical surface of the lens. All surfaces are carefully rubbed dry,
after which the lens is then ready for use.

It should be noted that the refractive indices of Canada balsam and glass are almost equal, so that when the lens is fixed to the cover slip we are in fact replacing the not absolutely plane surface of the lens by the plane surface of the cover slip. The lens thus obtained gives a good image and may be used successfully in the caps.

Round glass cover slips are used in the construction of some caps. It is difficult to work with a single glass cover slip because of its fragility. A better plan is to work with several cover slips at once, glued together with Canada balsam. In this case, the work can be done by hand, using fine-grain emery paper. The emery paper is wrapped around a soft pad to avoid excessive friction, which may place too great a strain on the glass. A paper pattern (a round piece of paper of the required diameter) is glued to the outer surface of one of the cover slips, and the glass is ground down to this size.

An important detail of many of the adaptors is the very thin piece of frosted glass which can easily be made from ordinary frosted glass in any optical workshop. It may also be made by the experimenter himself in the following manner. First, frosted glass of the required size is fixed by liquid Canada balsam to half a glass slide. To the other half of the glass slide is glued a rubber or wooden block shaped to serve as a handle by which the material may be held during the work, and the frosted glass is then ground on emery paper to the required thickness. First coarse, and then very fine, emery paper is used. The emery paper is backed by a smooth, hard surface. It should take the experimenter no more than 20-30 minutes to grind the frosted glass.

Making some of the very small components from glass calls for microtechniques of glass blowing, which differ slightly from ordinary glass blowing methods. Three types of heating apparatus are used: the ordinary alcohol or gas burner, a miniature alcohol burner, and a platinum wire heated to incandescence by an electric current. The burner in the miniature alcohol lamp is a long thin metal tube holding a cotton wick. The tube is usually several centimeters long and 1 mm in diameter. The end of the tube is placed horizontally so that the glass can be heated by placing it not only above the flame but also below it. The diameter of the flame from such a burner does not exceed 2-3 mm. If the platinum wire is being used it also is placed in such a position that the glass can be brought near to it both above and below. The benefits gained by this arrangement of the heating system will be clear to the experimenter as soon as he begins to take up microglass blowing. In many cases microglass blowing operations should not be done by hand; it is better to employ some type of simple micromanipulator. For example, to bend a very thin glass capillary tube to a right angle, it is held with one end in a micromanipulator, and the whole capillary tube is placed in a strictly horizontal position. Next, by the screws of the micromanipulator, the capillary tube is brought smoothly up to the incandescent platinum wire from below. In this way the wire and the capillary tube are perpendicular to each other. For a short distance from the platinum, a small segment of the capillary tube becomes soft and bends evenly under the weight of the unfixed part of the capillary tube. Within a few seconds the capillary tube is bent to a right angle. This operation is much more difficult by hand. One wrong movement or tremor of the hand and the capillary tube will be exposed to too high a temperature, or worse, will touch the platinum. In the first case, although the capillary tube does bend, it melts and the lumen is closed. In the second case, it melts immediately, sticks to the platinum wire, and is converted into a glass drop. Microglass blowing techniques demand from the experimenter knowledge of the fundamentals of glass blowing and the ability to use simple micromanipulators.

For some experiments, diaphragms with apertures ranging from 10 to 70 μ are introduced into the light source. Such diaphragms are easily made from ordinary foil. Foil is placed on a sheet of glass and gently pierced with a sharp-pointed needle. The hole thus made is measured and examined under a microscope or binocular loupe, and if it is too large or too small the operation is repeated on a fresh piece of foil. Diaphragms with a very narrow slit (from 10 to 70 μ) are made from safety razor blades. The two halves of a blade are fixed by BF-2 glue to a metal mount, and before the glue has dried, the slit between them is made the correct width using a binocular loupe.

Nearly all adaptors are made of paper. At first glance this work would seem to be very simple. However, it is one thing to glue large pieces of paper together, but quite a different thing to glue an item composed of very small pieces. To simplify this work, it is a good idea to begin by soaking both sides of the paper with BF-2 glue, to allow it to dry hard, and only then to begin forming the constructional details. Paper previously soaked in BF-2 glue can be stuck together by means of a small brush soaked in alcohol. When the brush moistens the point of contact between two pieces of paper, the glue on the paper quickly dissolves and when it quickly dries it glues the paper firmly and accurately.

With this I conclude my short list of tips for the experimenter who wishes to make his own caps. Naturally I have omitted details of operations and methods well known in laboratory practice, with which the experimenter will be familiar.

CONCLUSIONS

Of all the many methods which have been used to record eye movements, only those which have proved most successful can now be justified. However, none of the methods which have proved successful can be regarded as universal and perfect in all respects.

Depending on the experimenter's aims, on the conditions under which he must carry out his experiment, and finally, on the capacity of the subject, he will select one of these methods.

Experiments recording eye movements during fixation on a point are best carried out with the P_1 and P_3 models, for they provide very accurate records.

If the experiment is to take some time, and highly accurate records are nevertheless required, contact lenses with mirrors affixed to them should be used. and the records made as with the P_1 and P_3 caps, i.e., by a reflected beam of light. If, however, for some reason or other, the subject's eyes must remain perfectly free during the experiment, electrooculographic recording is the recommended method, despite its low accuracy.

When the subject's eyes and head must remain completely free and simultaneous records of the head and eye movements are required, motion-picture photography should be used. In this case, even to produce results of low accuracy, complicated analysis of the experimental material is required.

For producing images stationary relative to the retina, it is best to use the P_6, P_7, and P_8 caps.

Chapter II

PERCEPTION OF OBJECTS STATIONARY
RELATIVE TO THE RETINA

It has now been established that the provision of optimal working conditions for the eye requires some degree of constant (interrupted or continuous) movement of the retinal image.

This distinctive feature of the human eye was first noted by Adrian (1928). It was later concluded (Ditchburn and Ginsborg, 1952; Riggs et al., 1953) that objects stationary relative to the retina cannot be seen by an observer all the time. Finally, it was demonstrated by the use of the cap method (Yarbus, 1956g) that in any test field, unchanging and stationary relative to the retina, all visible differences disappear after 1-3 sec, and do not reappear in these conditions. The fact that in similar experiments previous authors did not observe permanent disappearance of visible differences may be explained by imperfections of their technique (incomplete stabilization of the retinal image).

In many animals, impulses run along the optic nerve in the main only in response to a change in the light acting on the retina. If impulses are regarded as carriers of information, it may be claimed that in most animals the process of vision quickly comes to an end when the retinal image is unchanged and stationary. On the other hand, the suggestion has been made that in man the absence of change and movement of the retinal image leads to the disappearance or to a sharp reduction in the number of the impulses transmitted from the eye to the central portion of the visual system. Later I shall use this as a working hypothesis, clearly recognizing that it has not yet been proved because no records have ever been made of human optic-nerve impulses.

In most experiments, the subject's second eye (the eye not directly participating in the experiment) was covered with a black bandage not allowing light to pass. In describing such experiments, I shall not mention the second eye. Cases when the subject looked at a fixation point with his second eye during the experiment or when the second eye was illuminated with light of some kind will be examined separately. In nearly every case, I shall give the type of cap used in the experiment. This will make it easier to understand the experiment, but does demand from the reader knowledge of the construction and function of each type of cap.

Objects whose images remain stationary on the retina whatever movement the eye makes are conventionally known as a "stationary test field." Objects whose images, as a result of movement of the objects themselves or of the eye, are displaced on the retina are conventionally called a "mobile test field." For example, when working with the type P_6 cap, in which a short-focus lens is used, the stationary test field is the image of the frosted glass of the cap, together with objects situated in its background and rigidly connected with the lens; another stationary test field is the dark background surrounding the frosted glass. A mobile test field in this case may be an object moving inside the cap, in front of the frosted glass, or the shadow of an object situated between the frosted glass and the light source, and moving across the background of the frosted glass.

When working with the type P_8 cap in which, besides a lens, a diaphragm with an aperture is used, the stationary test field is the screen or the several screens firmly fixed to the cap. The whole of the objectively stationary background whose image is displaced over the retina as a result of movement of the eyes may serve as a mobile test field. In addition, just as in the experiment with the P_6 cap, an object moving over the background of the screen may be used as a mobile test field.

A stationary and unchanging test field in which all visual contours have disappeared for the subject may be termed an "empty field" arising in artificial conditions.

Often as a result of fixation on a large and uniform enough surface, conditions of constant illumination arise within the retinal image of this surface. If the constancy of illumination lasts more than 2–3 seconds, the inner part of such a surface may be called an "empty field" arising in natural conditions.

1. FORMATION OF AN EMPTY FIELD

In a large series of experiments with the P_6 cap, the subjects were shown different stationary and unchanged test fields for perception, each of which occupied the whole field of vision of the eye. The test fields differed in their angular dimensions, shape, color, and contrast between details. The maximal visible brightness of the frosted glass of the cap was 3000 apostilbs,* when the diameter of the aperture of the diaphragm was 1-2 mm.

The first question to be answered was: does an empty field always appear in these conditions, i.e., do all visual contours disappear? The experiments showed that in every case, 1-3 seconds from the beginning of the experiment and after removal of all light of varying intensity passing through the sclera, all visual contours disappeared from the subject's field of vision. These contours did not reappear until the end of the experiment, i.e., for several minutes (unless something happened to disturb the constancy and strict immobility of the retinal image). The color of the empty field remained unchanged. Usually the subject will call this color "black," "dark grey," "dark," or "twilight," as when the eyes are closed.

These results have led certain investigators to consider that the empty field should be called black. However, this immediately raises the question: what does the observer see if, after an empty field has been formed, a black object moves against its background? Since the object moves, it must be visible, but a black object cannot be seen against a black background (if in fact it is black). To solve this problem, a series of experiments was carried out using the P_6 caps. The test field was a bright white circle surrounded by a black diaphragm with which it merged after the formation of the empty field. It was found that when a black object moved across the background of an empty field, the observer saw the object as black (much blacker than the empty field) and realized that it was a mistake to describe the empty field as black. Later experiments showed that an object of any color, moving across the background of an empty field, can be distinguished from the color of this field. These results showed that the subjective description of the color of the empty field (occupying the whole field of vision of the eye) is always conventional, for by direct comparison it is distinguished from any other color. The problem of the color of the empty field will be examined below.

If the cap were slightly displaced during the experiment (because of accidental contact with the eyelid or by a deliberate gentle tap) all the contours of the test field reappeared instantaneously. If the bandage was removed from the subject's second eye during the experiment and he opened this eye for perception, the character of the perception was just as if the eye to which the cap was fixed had been closed.

*Editors note: This is equivalent to a luminance of 300 millilamberts.

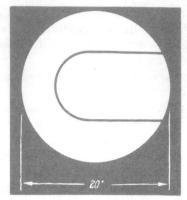

Fig. 32. Scheme of stationary test field. The filament of an incandescent lamp seen by the
subject through an aperture in a diaphragm fixed near the lamp.

The process of formation of the empty field and the field itself are
extremely sensitive to the slightest disturbances of the strict immobility or constancy of the retinal image. Attention is particularly
drawn to the possibility that light may enter the eye through the sclera.
Even if this light is constant, the illumination of the retina is fluctuating
because of the constant movements of the eye. It is therefore essential
to watch that during the experiment the bright beam of light falling on
the frosted glass of the cap does not illuminate the sclera. That is
why the modification in the construction of the adaptor for the P_6 cap,
which I have described, was introduced; this allows the frosted glass
of the cap to be illuminated from the nasal side, thus leaving the sclera
in almost complete darkness.

2. PERCEPTION OF VERY BRIGHT OBJECTS STATIONARY RELATIVE TO THE RETINA

In the experiments described in the previous section, the test
fields were of low or average luminance. It was important to verify
whether the differences in the stationary and constant test field disappeared if isolated parts of the field are very bright, almost blinding.

To investigate this problem, a special adaptor was made for the P_6
cap. This adaptor included a small electric lamp connected to a source
of current by very thin wires. The adaptor was placed in such a
position that the lens of the P_6 apparatus gave a sharp image of the
lamp filament on the retina. The image of this stationary test field is
shown schematically in Fig. 32. The thickness of the lamp filament

subtended a visual angle of 15 minutes. The brightness of the filament could be changed during the experiment by changing the voltage of
the supply. Most of the lamp was covered with black paper, so that no
light from it fell on the sclera, and when the experiments were carried
out in a dark room there was thus no possibility of light entering the
eye through the sclera. The wires supplying the lamp were so placed
that they did not interfere with the eye movement or displace the cap
on the eye. Before the experiments the subject received atropine to
dilate the pupil and immobilize the iris. To reduce eye movement, the
subject was given a fixation point for his free eye.

The experiments with this adaptor showed that when the elements
of the stationary test field are of dazzling brightness, all visual
contours disappear from the field. During the experiment the incandescent filament of the lamp disappeared for the subject 1-3 seconds
after the test field had become strictly constant and stationary. In
these circumstances the subject saw only the point fixated by the second
eye. If the lamp was switched off after the empty field had developed,
a transient appearance of the lost contours reappeared briefly, the
filament of the lamp appearing to be of dazzling brightness.

The results of the experiments described in sections 1 and 2 of this
chapter lead to the following conclusion: if a test field (of any size,
color, or brightness) becomes and remains strictly constant and stationary relative to the retina, then all contours in the field will disappear after 1-3 seconds and will not reappear.

I claim that the contours in the test field do not reappear because
their disappearance lasts for the duration of the experiment, i.e., for
several minutes. In addition, I am taking into consideration the results
of the experiment described in section 4 of Chapter I. I recall, for
example, the experiment in which the vessels of his own eye become
visible to an observer during oscillatory movements of a point source
of light, i.e., when the shadows of the blood vessels situated close to
the retina are in motion. If the movement of the light source stops,
the vessels disappear within 1-2 seconds and do not reappear as long
as the light source remains stationary.

The method generally believed to create a stationary retinal image,
using a contact lens with a mirror attached to it (see section 12 of
Chapter I), has not allowed experimenters to obtain lasting disappearance of contours from a test field. Usually the contours have disappeared for a few seconds, reappeared for a few seconds, and then
disappeared again. Because of these findings, certain authors are
doubtful that the contours of a stationary object can disappear for
any considerable time. The experiments I have just mentioned, es-

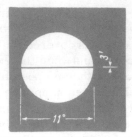

Fig. 33. Scheme of the stationary test field. The black thread is seen by the subject against the background of the frosted glass of the cap through a round hole in the diaphragm.

pecially those with the cap, have shown that the constant appearance of contours of the stabilized image during work with the contact lens can be attributed only to incomplete stabilization of the retinal image, a defect making the work of experimenters extremely difficult, and often making definite conclusions impossible.

This repeated disappearance of visible contours of a stationary test field (or sharp reduction in the resolving power of the eye) has been reported by many authors (Ditchburn and Ginsborg, 1952; Riggs et al., 1953; Ditchburn and Fender, 1955; Krauskopf, 1957; Ditchburn et al., 1959; Ditchburn and Pritchard, 1960; Clowes, 1961; Ditchburn, 1961). The important feature so far as we are concerned is that the results of all the investigations mentioned above confirm the important role of eye movements in vision.

3. PERCEPTION OF OBJECTS OF VARYING LUMINANCE STATIONARY RELATIVE TO THE RETINA

In this section an attempt is made to establish the minimal changes in the intensity of a light source at which a subject begins to see contours in a test field when the field is constantly stationary. The use of the P_6 cap ensured that the test field was stationary.

The stationary test field consisted of a round hole in a piece of black paper, intersected by a thin black silk thread. The subject saw the hole and the thread against the background of the frosted glass of the adaptor under angles indicated on Fig. 33.

The luminance of the test field (a circle) at which the subject looked through the diaphragm of the cap, 1.5 mm in diameter, was measured in apostilbs.

The frosted glass of the cap was illuminated with a beam of light from an incandescent lamp. The illuminance of the frosted glass was varied (either increased or diminished) linearly with time by means of a wedge placed between the light source and the cap. This adjustment was made by a rotating disc with a wedge-shaped slit. The rate of change in illuminance of the test field could be regulated by changing the speed of rotation of the disc. By changing the speed of movement of the wedge, the experimenter could produce the necessary change in luminance of the test field.

For any initial luminance of the test field l_0 it was easy to select rates of change of its luminance for which the subject saw the test field for a certain period of time clearly or very weakly, or did not see it at all. In these circumstances the interval during which the test field was seen was found to be a fraction of a second or might even exceed one second. With a low enough value of dl/dt, it had the appearance of a hardly detectable circle, the visual brightness of which increased with an increase in the value of dl/dt, after which the individual parts of the thread and, finally, the whole thread showed up against its background. When the subject reported the appearance of all contours in the test field, the phase during which he distinguished only certain parts of the thread against the background of the circle (the thread as a whole had not yet appeared) corresponded to a rate of change of luminance of the test field which I conventionally call "the threshold speed."

Knowing the initial luminance of the test field (l_0), the time of movement of the wedge (t), and the final luminance (l), the rate of change of luminance, i.e., dl/dt, could always easily be determined. In fact, since the luminance varied linearly with time, it was always true that $(l - l_0)/dt - dl/dt$.

Evidently when the pupil remains unchanged, the retinal illuminance (H) and its variation (dH/dt) bear a linear relationship to the corresponding luminances of the test field and to their variation.

As pointed out above, contours within the test field, in response to a variation of its luminance, were not noticed instantaneously by the subject but after a certain time lag (a fraction of a second). This time will be denoted subsequently by the Greek letter τ. Preliminary experiments showed that the value of τ is not constant but depends primarily on the value of $(dH/dt)/H$. However, I shall not examine this question in detail.

Most of the measurements were made on two subjects. First I attempted to discover how the appearance of contours in the test field depended on the direction (the sign) of the change of luminance of this field. The experiment showed that if a test field of a certain arbitrary luminance (l_0) changed into an empty field as a result of its immobility

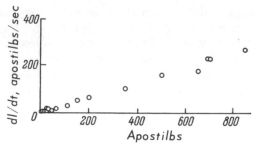

Fig. 34. Graph showing relationship between threshold rate of change of luminance of a test field dI/dt and the luminance (I_0) of this field.

relative to the retina, it reappeared for the subject when the luminance was either increased or decreased. The threshold rates were approximately equal in their absolute value for an increase and a decrease in luminance. During an increase in luminance the color of the circle appeared orange to the subject; during a decrease it appeared bluish or even blue.

Later an attempt was made to determine whether the threshold speed of change in luminance (from a constant I_0) depends on a series of conditions preceding the measurement—for example, whether it changes as a result of the preliminary action of a constant, bright light, or as a result of dark adaptation. The experiments showed that at the time the measurement was taken, i.e., 30–40 seconds after the formation of the empty field, these conditions had no significant effect on the magnitude of the threshold rate.

The aim of the following experiments was to study how the magnitude of the threshold rate of change of luminance depends on the initial luminance of the test field (I_0). The results of these experiments are given in Fig. 34. This figure shows that over the range of luminances from several apostilbs to 1000 (the diameter of the hole in the diaphragm was 1.5 mm), a linear relationship exists between these values. As the luminance I_0 increases, the threshold rate of change of luminance dI/dt increases proportionately. This result corresponds to the Weber-Fechner law. It follows from the foregoing remarks that the ratio between the threshold rate and the absolute luminance of this field is constant, i.e.,

$$\text{threshold } (dI/dt)/I_0 = \text{constant}$$

The values of these constants are shown in Fig. 35. In the present case these ratios, as the graph clearly shows, were approximately equal to 0.3 $\sec^{-1}$. This means that the contours in a test field stationary relative to the retina begin to be perceived by the subject when the luminance of this field changes at the rate of 30% per second. This figure remains constant throughout the full range of investigated luminances of the test field.

The value of the threshold rate thus determined may appear to be contrary to everyday experience, for we can detect changes in luminance taking place much more slowly than at the rate of 30% per second. However, the contradiction is only apparent, for we are discussing completely different processes. Under ordinary conditions of observation, the illuminance of individual elements of the retina is continually changing as a result of eye movement, regardless of whether, and at what rate, the luminance of the observed object changes. The figure of 30% per second is the rate of change of illuminance of an element of the retina at which signals appear in the corresponding nerve fiber. The changes in the luminance of objects which we perceive depends on how different these signals are when they have already appeared.

It was next found that when the ratio $(dI/dt)/I_0 = 1 \ \text{sec}^{-1}$, after a period of time τ, the subject saw the test field perfectly clearly (a thread with a thickness of three minutes of angle was seen absolutely clearly). In these circumstances this ratio remained unchanged for the whole range of investigated luminances (from several to 1000 apostilbs).

Bearing in mind that, with the pupil unchanged, the illuminance and the change in the illuminance of the retinal image bear a linear relationship to the luminance and the change in luminance of the test field, that through the investigated range of luminances the contours in the test field were clearly seen by the subject when

$$(dI/dt)/I_0 = (dH/dt)/H_0 = 1 \ \text{sec}^{-1}$$

and that

$$(dH/dt)/H = d\ln H/dt \,,$$

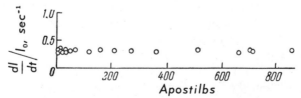

Fig. 35. Graph showing relationship between the ratio $(dI/dt)/I_0$ and luminance (I_0) of the test field, where dI/dt is the threshold rate of change in luminance of the test field.

the result obtained may be written in the form of the equation:

$$d \ln H/dt = 1 \text{ sec}^{-1}$$

Consequently, when the absolute value of the derivative of the natural logarithm of the illuminance in relation to time becomes and remains larger than unity ($d \ln H/dt > 1 \text{ sec}^{-1}$), after a certain interval τ the subject clearly sees that particular (Fig. 33) test field stationary relative to the retina.

In the present case (Fig. 33), the light circle began to appear at slower speeds than the thread, but in both cases the relationship $(dH/dt)/H_0 = \text{const}$ holds good. On this basis it may be concluded that this relationship will always be observed, even though the threshold speed may differ from one case to another.

If the change in illuminance takes place smoothly and over a long period $(> \tau)$, but $d \ln H/dt$ is constant, the corresponding element of the test field will become visible when $d \ln H/dt \geq \text{const}$. If, on the other hand, the change in H occupies a time τ_1, which is small in comparison with τ, the degree of visibility of the element will be determined, not by $d \ln H/dt$, but by $\Delta H/H$, i.e., by the extent to which H has changed.

4. PERCEPTION OF FLICKERING OBJECTS STATIONARY RELATIVE TO THE RETINA

The experiments suggest that vision is possible only when light of varying luminance or spectral composition acts on the elements of the retina. We shall now try to discover to what extent these conditions are not only essential, but also adequate.

Usually, in the process of vision, the image of the object is constantly moving over the retina as a result of eye movement. Because of this, the illuminance of the elements of the retina changes. The question arises: does this movement of the retinal image itself play a role in the process of vision? Can we, by excluding this movement, provide good conditions for perception by using varying illuminance? It is well known that during a bright flash of light, a person can detect many of the details and shades of color of an object. In these circumstances the duration of the flash may be so short that the corresponding retinal image must be practically stationary relative to the retina, and consequently, the eye movement cannot have taken part in the process of vision. In addition, the facts described in the preceding section show that the eye notices very small details of a stationary test field if its luminance varies sufficiently in the course of a short enough time.

However, a single flash or a single change in the luminance of a stationary test field (when dI/dt retains its sign) cannot provide satisfactory conditions for perception. In the first case the subject has insufficient time, and in the second the color of the stationary test field is distorted, with either increase or particularly, decrease in luminance. For this reason, to facilitate the perception of a stationary test field, the last possibility was used, illumination of the field with flickering light.

In most experiments the visual test object was the test field shown schematically in Fig. 36. Pieces of completely opaque black film, a sharp image of which was seen by the subject against the bright frosted glass, were fixed to a very thin glass cover slip placed in a P_6 cap. Sometimes, instead of black film, brightly colored gelatin (transparent) films were used. In all cases the diameter of the test field, i.e., of the bright round background, was 17°.

The flicker frequency varied from 1 to 50 cycles. During each cycle light and darkness were equal in duration. Each increase of the light to a maximum and decrease to complete darkness took not more than 0.005 sec. The luminance of the frosted glass of the cap was 3000 apostilbs. The diameter of the artificial pupil (the diaphragm of the cap) was 1 mm.

First an attempt was made to discover how the resolving power of the eye changes with a change in the frequency of the flicker on the frosted glass of the cap when the test field (illustrated in Fig. 36) is strictly stationary relative to the retina, and the sclera is in total darkness.

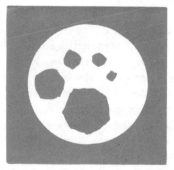

Fig. 36. Scheme of a stationary test field. Five black spots seen by the subject against a background of the frosted glass of the cap; the angular diameter of the hole in the diaphragm (the bright circle) is 17°; the diameters of the black spots are 6, 4, 2, 1.5, and 1°, respectively.

It was found that so long as the flicker frequency did not exceed four cycles, the subject observed all the black spots against the background of the flickering circle. When the flicker frequency was five cycles, the subject could no longer detect the smallest black spot (with a diameter of 1°). It had become pale and was indistinguishable from the flickering field. With flicker of six cycles, the subject observed only the largest or the two largest spots of the test field (with diameters of 6 and 4°). With flicker at the rate of 7–9 cycles, the subject no longer saw any of the dark spots on the test field, and saw only the light flickering circle (diameter 17°). When the flicker frequency was 10–11 cycles, the subject again began to see the two largest (sometimes the three largest) spots, but as the critical flicker frequency was approached, they again disappeared. At the critical flicker frequency (in this case about 30 cycles), the circle disappeared, and the whole field of vision became an empty field.

The following conclusions may be drawn from the results of these experiments: first, with an increase in the frequency of the flickering light the details of the test field, stationary relative to the retina, do not all disappear at once as the flicker frequency increases—the smaller details are the first to disappear; second, a range of flicker frequencies (7–9 cycles) exists in which the resolving power of the eye is at its lowest (disregarding the region close to the critical flicker frequency); when the flicker frequency is above the critical level, an empty field appears just as during continuous illumination. In every case (whatever the flicker frequency), the resolving power of the eye was much below normal.

In the first series of experiments the sclera was in total darkness. Let us now consider how illumination of the sclera influences the results of the same experiments, when the light falling on the frosted glass and that falling on the sclera flicker synchronously.

In this experiment, the part of the light beam not falling directly on the frosted glass of the cap was utilized (the beam of light directed towards the frosted glass was always wider than the glass). By placing a sheet of white paper on the subject's temple, an illuminated screen was obtained, scattered light from which fell on the sclera and flickered synchronously with the flicker on the test field.

In these conditions, the black spots of the test field began to disappear more quickly and at rather lower flicker frequencies. With a frequency of 7–9 cycles, when the screen was moved so close to the eye that the sclera was well illuminated with scattered flickering light, not only the black spots of the test field disappeared, but also the 17° bright circle itself. The subject saw only the flickering light and could detect none of the details in the visual field. The light reflected from the paper and falling on the sclera was no brighter than the light falling on the sclera in the room from the ordinary daylight or artificial light. These results suggest that with adequate brightness of scattered light, in the conditions described above, the eye becomes incapable of perceiving any details in a test field.

Further experiments were carried out to determine the resolving power of the eye when a flickering light is suddenly switched on (after complete darkness), and to ascertain its changes in time if the flicker frequency remains constant.

In these experiments, the flicker frequency was 8 cycles. The flickering light was switched on or off by a shutter fixed to the light source. When the flickering light was switched on, the subject saw all elements of the test field sharply. The circle appeared white, with a noticeably yellowish hue, and the black spots appeared black. Next, for several seconds, the black spots gradually become paler and disappeared on the flickering circle. When the flickering light was switched off, the subject saw the usual after-image: for a period of 1-2 seconds the circle appeared black, with a noticeably bluish tinge, while the black spots looked grey and much lighter than the background. These results suggest that if the retinal image is stationary, a single illumination of the object, even for a short time, allows the eye (depending on the luminance and duration of illumination) to resolve the small elements of the object. Periodic repetition of the same type of illumination (particularly at certain frequencies) will cause a sharp decrease in the resolving power of the eye.

In the next series of experiments, the effect of constant illumination on the resolving power of the eye was studied in conditions when the test field flickered at frequency of 5 cycles. Before the light was switched on, the subject usually saw at least four black spots against the background of the flickering circle. Illumination was provided by a bright beam of light, directed at the required moment to the exposed part of the sclera (in these circumstances orange light scattered by the sclera fell on the retina).

In these experiments, the subject perceived a flash of orange light when the constant illumination was switched on. If the illumination was very bright, all the details of the test field disappeared at once (sometimes even the sensation of flicker disappeared). This was followed by the appearance of the flickering background and the larger spots (three or four) of the test field. In every case after the light was switched on, the black details were distinctly orange in color and the flickering circle appeared bluish. By comparison with the moment before illumination, the resolving power of the eye was slightly lower (it fell as the intensity of illumination increased). Switching off the light was perceived at once as an improvement in the resolving power of the eye. All five black spots were seen on a white circle, and after a few seconds, the 1° spot again disappeared.

In one experiment an attempt was made to determine the effect of the brightness of the flickering light on the resolving power of the eye when the test field remained stationary and the flicker frequency constant (5 cycles). These experiments showed that any increase beyond a certain luminance of flicker was accompanied by a decrease in the resolving power of the eye. The black spots of the test field became lighter, and the visual contrast between spots and background diminished.

Evidently, as the luminance of the flicker increased, the amount of light scattered by the optical system of the cap and the eye also increased. In these circumstances, part of the scattered light fell on the retinal image of the black spots. When the scattered light falling on the retinal image of the black spots reached a certain level of brightness, it began to have the effect described earlier in the experiments in which the sclera was illuminated by flickering light. This evidently explains the decrease observed in the resolving power of the eye.

The color of the flickering light falling on the frosted glass of the cap was changed in a series of experiments with a stationary test field. This procedure did not produce any marked change in the resolving power of the eye.

When the flicker frequency dropped below 3-5 cycles, conditions frequently developed in which the test field appeared negative to the subject. The black spots appeared light against the background of a dark flickering circle. This phenomenon developed particularly frequently when the luminance of the flicker was reduced and when the light thrown on the frosted glass of the cap was a saturated blue color.

If, instead of black spots on a white background, transparent colored films were used, even with a high saturation and large angular dimensions (7-8°), they disappeared for the subject sooner and faster than the black opaque spots (in otherwise identical experimental conditions). The color of the flickering circle acquired the hue of the films occupying the greater part of the area of the circle. Switching off the flickering light (of different frequencies) led to the appearance of clear and saturated after-images.

In analogous tests made with the subject's second eye (without the cap) open, the elements of the test field invariably disappeared more rapidly and the resolving power of the eye was even further reduced.

This phenomenon was observed even when the subject fixated on a small fixation point in a completely darkened room with his free eye.

Use of a flickering light that changed smoothly from light to dark and from dark to light on the frosted glass had no significant effect on the experimental results.

In conclusion, we may mention again that when an empty field is filled with a flickering environment, a very important role is played by illumination of the retina with scattered light (light scattered by the sclera or even by the transparent media of the eye).

It is therefore clear that a constant (continuous or interrupted) movement of the retinal image is essential to ensure satisfactory working conditions for the human eye, and that this cannot be produced by any method of illuminating images stationary relative to the retina.

Ditchburn and Fender (1955) carried out experiments with a flickering image stationary relative to the retina. The test field was a flickering circle divided by a black line. These authors claim that the most favorable conditions for perception were obtained at the critical flicker frequency. These claims do not agree with my own findings but would appear to be attributable to the inadequacy of the methods used.

5. PERCEPTION OF OBJECTS OF CHANGING COLOR, STATIONARY RELATIVE TO THE RETINA

We shall now consider to what extent the apparent color appearing on an empty field during a change in illumination depends on this change and to what extent it depends on the color of the background (the originally empty field), against which this change takes place.

In the experiments the test field was the frosted glass visible to the subject in the P_6 cap against a black background. The frosted glass was rectangular, and its sides had angular dimensions of $14 \times 7°$. To the outer surface of the frosted glass were fixed two polaroids with mutually perpendicular planes of polarization. The border of contact between the polaroids divided the frosted glass into two squares. By directing light onto the frosted glass from two sources covered with filters and suitably oriented relative to the polaroids, the experimenter could change the color of the two halves of the test field independently and at will. The polarization planes of the polaroids on the frosted glass (perpendicular to each other) were parallel respectively to the polarization planes of the polaroids of the light sources, so that the color of each half of the test field was determined entirely by light from one source. In addition, nonpolarized light from a third source was thrown on to the frosted glass of the cap. By means of this third light source, the experimentor was able to add an equal amount of light to the two halves of the test field and then to modify it as necessary. Naturally, the changes in this light were always equal for the two halves of the test field.

The maximal luminance of the frosted glass of the cap did not exceed 3000 apostilbs when the diameter of the hole in the diaphragm was 1.5 mm. Let us assume that the color of one half of the test field was A, and that of the other half B. At a given moment, as a result of its immobility relative to the retina, the test field becomes empty. Now to both fields an equal addition of light C is made, subthreshold for both A and B, i.e., the colors A and B simultaneously become A' = A + C, and B' = B + C. This addition is made immediately after formation of the empty field, i.e., when the state of the eye has changed only slightly on account of adaptation. During this change in illumination, both fields must appear against the background of an empty field. If their color depends entirely on the differences between A' − A and B' − B, it must therefore depend entirely on C, and both fields must therefore appear to be always equal, whatever the nature of A, B, and C. Conversely, if the fields appearing after the addition of the third color to two different colors A and B are different, then however this difference might be expressed, it shows that the signal which is formed depends not only on the nature of the added color C, but also on the color to which the addition was made.

When the experiment is carried out in this way, it is very important that the subject be asked only one question: are the fields appearing after the addition the same or are they different? He must not be asked to evaluate this difference. Verbal descriptions of differences between two colors inevitably possess a subjective quality; the presence of a difference of some sort as a rule is a much more reproducible factor.

I shall describe an experiment (Fig. 37) in which one half of the test field was saturated red and the other half saturated green. After the test field had become an empty field, a beam of pale blue light was thrown in addition on both halves of the frosted glass. At the moment the blue light was switched on, the test field appeared to the subject to be a uniform blue color. Next, after a period of one to three seconds, this color disappeared and the empty field reappeared.

In actual fact, when the blue color was switched on, although the subject saw the test field as uniformly blue, the red half of the test field turned crimson and the green half bluish-green. Consequently, a great difference in color remained between the two halves although it was not perceived by the subject.

The following conclusion was drawn from experiments such as these on the discrimination between colors A, B, and C. Any sub-threshold (for A and B) increase in the light falling on an empty field reveals no differences in a test field if the experiment is carried out in conditions in which the state of the eye has not changed appreciably because of adaptation. At the moment the light is increased, the whole test field appears to be uniformly the color of the added color C. In other words, the color seen by the subject at the moment of an above-threshold increase in the light falling on the empty field is determined purely by this added light and is independent of the background against which this addition is made.

However, the facts described above are valid only for an increase in the intensity of illumination, but they do not hold good when the added light is removed, such as during the change from A' = A + C and B' = B + C to A and B. In this case ("negative addition"), both fields appeared different, and their color depended both on the initial colors A and B and on the added color C.

The results of a series of experiments in which the colors A, B, and C were changed were as follows. Any supra-threshold decrease in the light falling on the empty field revealed contours in the test field, but in these circumstances the visible color of the test field was distorted, i.e., it did not correspond to any of the colors A, B, and C.

These simple rules were verified for the different colors A, B, and C on several subjects, but one important reservation must be made. For a subject to see a certain change in brightness against the background of a test field, the change must be above a certain threshold itself, in accordance with the Weber-Fechner law, increases with the luminance of the test field. I showed earlier (in section 3 of this chapter) that changes in the luminance of the empty field essential for revealing differences in the test field also correspond to the Weber-Fechner law. Later I tried to observe this in conditions analogous to those just described; the experimental results were purely qualitative in character.

In these experiments A, B, and C had the same spectral composition but differed considerably in brightness. If the brightness of A was much greater than the brightness of B, the added brightness C was chosen to be above the threshold for B but below the threshold for A. In this case, when the addition C was switched both on and off, only the less bright field appeared. This perfectly natural result qualifies the conclusion that during the positive addition, the fields to which light is added remain indistinguishable. For this reason, in describing the experiment, I have emphasized that the additions were deliberately chosen to be supra-threshold for both fields.

The threshold of visible changes of light depends on the background against which they take place. The important feature is that this relationship is maintained even when this background cannot be perceived by the subject because of its immobility relative to the retina.

In the next experiment I attempted to discover whether short flashes of light and short interruptions of light are perceived, and if so, how, under the conditions described at the beginning of this section. Let us assume that one half of the test field is color A and the other half color B. Next, after the appearance of an empty field, a flash of light is thrown over the whole field, as a result of which during the time of the flash the halves of the test field have the color $A' = A + C$ and $B' = B + C$. In all cases when the duration of the flashes lay between 0.01 and 0.05 sec, the subject did not notice the differences in the test field, and the apparent color of the flash appeared to be color C. When the duration of the flash reached 1 sec, differences again appeared between the two halves of the test field following a very short but perceptible interval of time after the light was switched off.

Let us now assume that one half of the test field is the color $A' = A + C$, and that the other half is the color $B' = B + C$. After development of an empty field, component C is switched off for a short period of time. In this series of experiments the exclusion of component C for some hundredths of a second was perceived by the subject only as some kind of change in color (he could not give the color a name). The exclusion of component C for several tenths of a second was perceived by the subject as flashes of light, in apparent color resembling supplementary color C. If component C was excluded for 1 sec, the subject then saw the difference between the two halves of the test field.

6. CHANGES IN THE STATE OF THE RETINA AFTER FORMATION OF AN EMPTY FIELD

When an empty field forms, all differences in color apparent to the subject gradually disappear until eventually the colors are indistinguishable. In the beginning this diminution of all visual contours resembles, at least externally, the familiar phenomenon of adaptation developing when the eye fixates on a colored object of one color against the background of another color. As a result of adaptation, even with slight eye movement, the apparent colors of the object become paler (lose their saturation) and closer together. Admittedly, this process, when observed without the cap, takes place much more slowly than formation of an empty field; indeed, it hardly ever progresses to the complete disappearance of visual contours. But the evident similarity between the two phenomena has led many investigators to apply the term "adaptation" to both processes. Originally, I also considered these phenomena to be identical, but I was puzzled by the great difference in speed of the changes observed. For this reason, I wondered whether the process of adaptation ends when an empty field forms or whether it continues after the field is formed.

The P_6 cap was used in this series of experiments. The stationary test field was a light rectangle on a black background (the rectangular piece of frosted glass). The height of the rectangle was 20° and its width 10°, and the color of the black background remained constant. The color of the rectangle was changed by means of filters.

In the first series of experiments in which different filters were used, the bottom half of the rectangle, acting as stationary test field, was shielded by black paper opaque to light before each experiment. Initially, the subject saw a bright square against a black background (the top half of the rectangle), but an empty field developed after 1-3 sec. For the subject, the bright square was merged with the background. The subject remained in this state for 1-2 min, after which the black paper was removed carefully from the bottom half of the rectangle so as not to disturb the immobility of the image. The subject saw a bright square for 1-3 sec (the bottom half of the rectangle), after which the square again appeared to merge with the dark background, i.e., an empty field developed when both halves of the rectangle had the same intensity of illumination. The light was switched off after 2-3 sec, and the subject saw two quite different after-images, belonging to the top and bottom halves of the rectangle.

In one of the experiments, shown schematically in Fig. 38, the rectangle acting as stationary test field was screened by a red filter and, in addition, its bottom half was covered with a neutral filter absorbing 85% of the light. Initially, the subjects saw a red rectangle, the top half of which was much brighter than the bottom half. Subsequently (after 1-3 sec) an empty field appeared (both halves of the rectangle merged with the black background), and the subject remained in this state for 2 min. At the end of this period, the red and neutral filters were removed at the same time, with care taken not to disturb the immobility of the retinal image, and the rectangle was illuminated with white light. After this change, the subject saw the rectangle reappear as pale blue (a shade similar to the added color) and

consisting of two sharply different halves. The top half of the rectangle, i.e., the half illuminated previously by the brighter red light,
appeared bluer and darker than the bottom half. In these new experimental conditions the rectangle again disappeared after 1–3 sec, i.e.,
an empty field again developed. Immediately after this, the light was
completely switched off and an after-image appeared, a dark blue
rectangle, also consisting of two sharply different halves, but this
time the top half appeared lighter than the bottom half.

Similar results are obtained with filters other than the red.
Naturally, the color added will be complementary to the other color.

We may conclude from these experiments that two different processes exist: the first is a "fast" process of disappearance of all contours
in the stationary test field, and the second a "slow" easily demonstrated process—by means of after-images, for example. The next
experiment was undertaken to make long and continuous observations
on the slow process.

A red filter made of gelatin film was placed between the frosted
glass but did not touch it. It was big enough to cover the whole visual
field whatever movements the eye made. Since movements of the filter
could not be seen by the eye through the frosted glass, they could not
prevent the formation of an empty field. A hole was punched in the
gelatin film, through which a beam of white light fell on the rectangular
frosted glass, and as a result of continuous movement of the eye, the
subject saw this beam the whole time as a light spot (Fig. 39). Movement of this spot in the field of vision did not prevent the appearance
of an empty field. The empty field appeared 1–3 sec after the beginning
of the experiment. When the empty field first appeared, the spot
was seen as a bright white against a dark grey background. Then,
because of the slow process, for a period of 30–40 sec the apparent
color of the spot changed appreciably; at the end of this period it
was a saturated blue. Similar results were obtained with filters of any
other color. The spot, white when the empty field first appeared, later
acquired a saturated color approximately complementary to the color
of the stationary test field. The results of these experiments suggest that after the appearance of an empty field the action of constant
stimuli stationary relative to the retina substantially alters the state
of the retina—the magnitude and character of its reaction to the same
radiation are modified. The slow process is not observed by the
subject after appearance of the empty field, since there are no signals
in the optic nerve. When a signal appears, it is influenced by the state
of the retina, modified as a result of the slow process.

7. PERCEPTION OF OBJECTS STATIONARY RELATIVE TO THE RETINA AND OCCUPYING PART OF THE VISUAL FIELD

This section describes experiments in which the subject's eye perceived stationary and mobile test fields simultaneously.

For these experiments a P_8 cap was used, fitted with screens (stationary test field) of different colors and sizes. Usually the screen consisted of two halves of different colors, most frequently black and white. The background (mobile test field) against which the screens were seen consisted in some cases of a plain sheet of paper (all of one color), and in other cases of a colored mosaic—a sheet of cardboard with pictures from Ostwald's color atlas glued to it.

Just as in the preceding experiments, all visual contours within the stationary test field disappeared within 1–3 sec after the experiment began, and it became a visually homogeneous empty field. The apparent color of the moving test field did not change. When the angular dimensions of the stationary test field were less than those of a solid-color moving test field, and the first field lay within the second, the apparent color of the empty field merged within a few seconds with the color of the moving test field. In other words, if the shutter of the cap was wholly against the background of a sheet of paper all one color and uniformly illuminated, the shutter regardless of color and size, merged after 1–3 sec with the background (the paper) and was not perceived by the subject, who saw only the sheet of paper (Fig. 10). In this case the empty field was analogous to the blind spot, which was also filled with the color of the surrounding background.

In one experiment the subject transferred his gaze from a sheet of red paper to a sheet of blue paper, so that the round shutter, consisting of black and white halves, was seen against first one sheet and then the other. Immediately after the change of background the apparent color of the shutter changed within a few seconds from red to blue when the gaze was switched to the blue paper, and from blue to red when it was switched to the red paper.

In other words, subjectively, the color of the shutter always changed to that of the uniform background, merging with it completely within a few seconds. In fact, of course, the color of the black-and-white shutter remained unchanged but, as the experiments showed, played no part in this case. This confirms the earlier hypothesis that signals from the part of the retina corresponding to the empty field, particularly to the empty field of the shutter, do not reach the optic nerve.

If the moving test field (the background) was a colored mosaic (pieces of paper of various colors glued to cardboard), and the stationary test field (the shutter) had a much larger visual angle than the uniform segments of the moving test field (the separate pieces of paper), the empty field could not merge with the background, and its apparent color remained permanently dark gray; when the other eye was illuminated, the empty field assumed the color of this illumination. If the stationary test field and the individual uniformly colored portions of the moving test field were approximately the same size, a constant tendency was observed for the apparent color of the empty field to merge with the background of the parts of the moving test field. Fusion was complete only when the empty field was entirely against the background of one of the uniformly colored parts of the moving test field.

In one experiment (Fig. 41), two identical black-and-white stationary test fields A_1 and A_2 (two shutters) were located a short distance apart against the background of a moving test field B_1 and B_2. The diameter of each stationary test field was $10°$. The distance between the edges of these fields was $10°$. The moving test field consisted of two halves (B_1 and B_2). One half (B_1) of the field was checkered, and consisted of different colored squares, each with a visual angle considerably smaller than $10°$. The second half of this field (B_2) was a solid color (a large sheet of red paper). The subject held his eyes in such a position that the stationary test field A_1 was always against the background of the checkered half of the moving test field (B_1), and the test field A_2 was against the uniformly colored background B_2. Our purpose was to discover what the apparent color of each empty field would be if, because of the experimental conditions, the apparent color of one of them could not merge with the checkered background of the moving test field B_1, but the apparent color of the other could merge with the uniform background B_2. In other words, is it possible, in certain conditions, to change the apparent colors of empty fields, separated in space, simultaneously yet independently?

Between 1 and 3 sec after the experiment began, the contours of the stationary test fields disappeared, and each became an empty field. The surface of these fields appeared to the subject to be a uniform dark gray. Immediately afterward, the apparent color of the empty field lying against the uniform background B_2 merged with the apparent color of this background. The apparent color of the empty field lying against the checkered background B_1 remained dark gray. When the second eye was illuminated in this experiment, the apparent color of the empty field lying against the checkered background changed, simultaneously with the color of the whole background (i.e., B_1 and B_2), to the color of the light illuminating the second eye. The empty field which had merged with the uniform background B_2 did not show up at all in these conditions.

In the last experiment of this series, the stationary test field was a black-and-white shutter seen by the subject against the background of a screen, a uniformly and identically illuminated sheet of red paper (Fig. 42). The shutter was 10° in diameter. Besides the diaphragm of the P_8 cap, through which the subject looked at the screen, a stop was fixed to the cap to restrict the field of vision, a second round diaphragm which left the central area of the retina (50°) free for perception. The sole purpose of restricting the visual field by this stop was so that during the experiment, with small movements of the eye, the edge of the screen (the edge of the sheet of red paper) did not fall within the subject's field of vision. During the first moment of the experiment the subjects saw a red circle (the central part of the screen) and a black-and-white shutter against its background.

A few seconds after the experiment began, an empty field developed over the whole field of vision, and the subject said that it had become dark. Since the screen was stationary, its image moved over the retina as the eye moved. However, since the edge of the screen did not fall within the field of vision (limited by the stop), and the screen itself was illuminated uniformly, the illuminance of all points of the retina was unchanged; this was equivalent to immobility of the retinal image.

Next moment, four narrow strips of white paper were fixed to the red screen to form a square situated inside the restricted field of vision. The size and position of the square were such that the shutter lay inside the square (within the field of vision), and with small eye movements the square did not touch the shutter).

The subject immediately noticed the strips of paper and the fact that the field restricted by these strips became red after a few seconds, i.e., adopted the true color of the screen. If the strips of paper were removed, the empty field again developed over the whole visual field, and after a few seconds the apparent color of the screen changed from red to gray; it merged with the color of the stop limiting the field of vision, and everything appeared dark to the subject. The important result of this experiment from our point of view was that the black-and-white shutter, having disappeared for the subject at the beginning of the experiment, did not subsequently reappear. The apparent color of the shutter always changed in step with the apparent color of the screen.

Important conclusions may be drawn from these results. First of all, the empty field clearly has no color of its own. No change in the luminance of any part of the field of vision disturbs the empty field bordering on this area. A change in the color of the region surrounding the empty field may modify the apparent color of the empty field within very wide limits.

Perception of the empty field cannot be identified with the perception arising in the absence of active light, i.e., the perception of a stationary black test field, before its conversion into an empty field, cannot be identified with perception of the empty field. A black color corresponds to a signal indicating absence of light, but an empty field corresponds to the absence of a signal. When a signal denoting absence of light, is present, we see black, but when no signal is present on an empty field we may see any color.

The general conclusion may be drawn from all the preceding experiments that in ordinary conditions of perception we are often concerned with empty fields arising in natural conditions, when we examine large surfaces of uniform color, for example a cloudless blue sky or a monochrome screen.

In fact, although the human eye is continually in movement, frequently these movements are within the limit of a limited solid angle. If a uniform background has angular dimensions greater than this solid angle, there must be a region of the retina within which no changes take place during a period of time sufficient for the formation of an empty field (1-3 sec). An empty field will develop under these conditions on the corresponding area of the perceived object, but it is subjectively imperceptible because it assumes the color of the surroundings. In perception of a uniform surface, the eye extrapolates the apparent color from the edges of a surface to its center. The absence of signals from a particular area of the retina provides the eye with information that this area corresponds to a uniform surface, the color of which does not change and is equal to the color of its edges. The change from the state of the first moment of perception, when the eye receives signals from the whole surface, to the state when extrapolation is used, takes place smoothly and in natural conditions is never perceived by the observer.

The apparent color of an empty field arising in natural conditions is always equal to the color of its borders, i.e., it is always equal to the color of the surface against which it arises.

The apparent color of the empty field arising in natural conditions is determined by one of two conditions. In the first case, the color depends on the color visible to the subject's second eye. When the

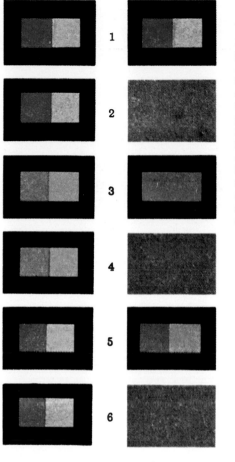

Fig. 37. Scheme of an experiment. In each pair of figures, a stationary test field is shown on the left, and the apparent color of this field on the right. 1) Test field and its apparent color at the beginning of the experiment; 2) after 1-3 sec an empty field appears and all visual contours disappear; 3) pale blue light added equally to the two halves of the test field (red and green). The subject sees only the added light on both halves of the field; 4) after 1-3 sec an empty field appears; 5) blue light switched off. The contours of the stationary test field are again apparent to some extent to the subject; 6) after 1-3 sec an empty field appears.

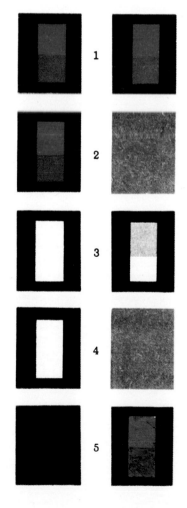

Fig. 38. Scheme of an experiment. In each pair of figures, the stationary test field is shown on the left and the apparent color of this field on the right. 1) Test field and its apparent color at the beginning of the experiment; 2) after 1-3 sec an empty field appears, and the eye remains in this state for 2 min; 3) after 2 min, the colored filters are removed, the test field becomes white. At this moment the subject sees the test field as consisting of two halves (the top half darker than the bottom); 4) after 1-3 sec an empty field again appears; 5) when the light falling on the frosted glass of the cap is totally switched off, the subject again sees the test field as consisting of two halves (the top half lighter than the bottom).

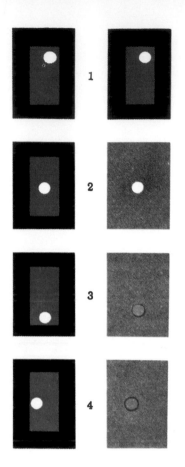

Fig. 39. Scheme of an experiment. In each pair of figures, the stationary test field and bright white object moving against the background of this field are shown on the left. The apparent color of the test field and object is shown in the right figure of each pair. 1) Test field and its apparent color at the beginning of the experiment; 2) after 1-3 sec an empty field appears (the object still appears white); 3) after 20 sec (the object appears blue); 4) the picture after 40 sec (the object appears dark blue).

Fig. 40. Scheme of an experiment. In each pair of figures, the one on the left shows a mobile test field against which is seen the stationary test field, a black-and-white screen. The apparent color of these fields is illustrated in the right-hand figure of each pair. 1) Test field and its apparent color at the beginning of the experiment; 2) after 1-3 sec an empty field is formed on the screen, and it merges with the mobile test field; 3) the screen against the border between the red and blue halves of the mobile test field.

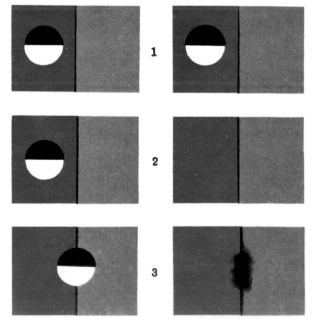

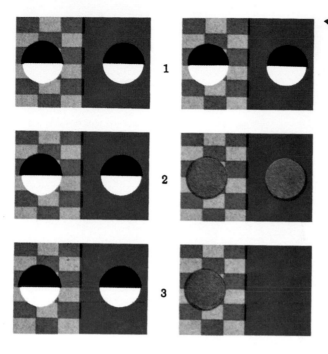

Fig. 41. Scheme of experiment. On the left in each pair of figures is shown the mobile test field on which are superimposed two stationary test fields, two black-and-white shutters rigidly affixed to the cap. One half of the mobile test field is checkered, and the other is of one color. The apparent color of the test field is shown on the right figure of each pair. 1) Test fields and their apparent color at the beginning of the experiment; 2) after 1-3 sec an empty field is formed on the shutters; 3) at the next moment the apparent color of the right shutter merges with the color of the uniform background. The apparent color of the left shutter cannot merge with the checkered background.

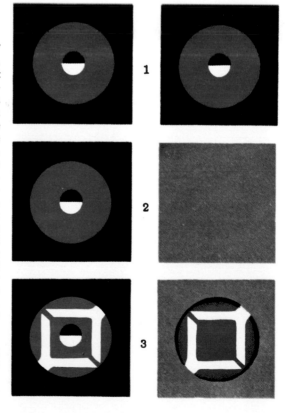

Fig. 42. Scheme of an experiment. In each pair of figures, the test field, consisting of a black diaphragm with a round aperture, a black-and-white shutter, and a solid red background, seen by the subject through the aperture in the diaphragm, is shown on the left. The diaphragm and shutter are rigidly attached to the cap (stationary test fields). The red background is the mobile test field. The apparent color of the test field is shown by the right figure in each pair. 1) Test field and its apparent color at the beginning of the experiment; 2) because of the uniformity of the red background and the immobility of the remaining parts of the test field, after 1-3 sec an empty field is formed inside the diaphragm; 3) when strips of white paper forming a square are placed on the red background, the apparent color of the background then becomes red, but the black-and-white shutter does not appear.

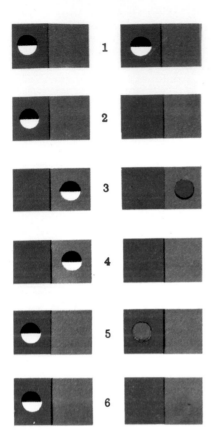

Fig. 43. Scheme of an experiment. In each pair of figures, the left one shows a red-and-blue mobile test field on which is a black-and-white shutter, the stationary test field. The apparent color of these fields is shown on the right figure of each pair. 1) Test field and its apparent color at the beginning of the experiment; 2) a few seconds later an empty field was formed on the shutter, and its apparent color merged with the color of the red half of the background; 3) when the points of fixation were changed so that the empty field was against the background of the blue half, for the first few seconds the apparent color of the empty field remained red; 4) then the apparent color of the empty field merged into the blue of the background; 5) after a second change of points of fixation for the first few seconds so that the empty field was against the red half of the background, the apparent color of the empty field remained blue; 6) then the apparent color of the empty field merged with the red of the background.

Fig. 44. Scheme of two experiments. The left column of figures shows stages in the disappearance of the shutter (stationary test field) against a background changing color slowly and smoothly. The even change in the background color prolongs the disappearance of the shutter and makes the process suitable for observation. The right column of figures shows stages in the appearance of the shutter under similar experimental conditions.

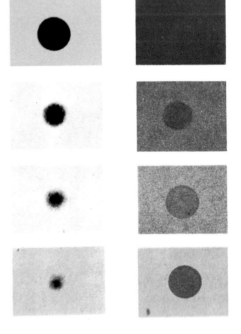

second eye is closed, the empty field is "dark," a dark gray background; when the second eye is illuminated, the background assumes the color of the illumination. The second case is observed when, in artificial conditions, the empty field lies on the background of a uniform surface and merges with this surface; in other words, the empty field arising on the shutter of the cap can assume the color of the empty field arising in natural conditions. This merger of fields can be understood if it is remembered that in both cases empty fields develop as a result of the absence of signals, and that the absence of signals from a given area of the retina is interpreted in the same way by the higher levels of the visual system. It can be said that the visual system "identifies" an empty field arising in artificial conditions with an empty field arising in natural conditions.

That is why, therefore, the empty field obtained by means of caps is always a uniform background (all visual contours with the field disappear), and the apparent color of the field is always the color of the surroundings, when it lies against a uniform surface. Hence the properties of an empty field arising in natural conditions may be studied in experiments with caps.

8. DELAY IN SEEING THE COLOR OF AN EMPTY FIELD

In this section we examine the delay experienced in seeing the color of an empty field.

The Γ_8 cap was used in all experiments. The stationary test field was a black-and-white shutter, the angular size of which was 10°. The mobile test field consisted of various paper screens.

In the first experiment, repeating one of the experiments in the previous section, the mobile test field was a paper screen, half red and half blue (Fig. 43). The essence of the experiment was that, after the appearance of an empty field on the shutter, the subject looked at each half of the screen in turn and chose his position so that the shutter was first entirely within the red half and then entirely within the blue half. When the empty field appeared on each half of the screen, it assumed the color of the half and merged with it completely. We have already observed this result.

The important feature of the present experiment was as follows. When the subject changed his points of fixation after appearance of the empty field on the red half so that it appeared against the blue half, the color of the empty field was still red (when first seen against the blue half), then, within a period of 2-3 sec, its color changed smoothly into blue, merging with the blue background. With the change from the blue half of the screen to the red, the empty field changed color to red in the same way and at the same speed and merged with the red background.

In all the subsequent experiments of this series, the shutter (stationary test field) was directed by the subject to the center of a white screen and remained in that position until the end of that experiment. By means of two light sources, camera shutters, and a system of rotating polaroids in a dark room, the experimenter changed the color of the screen (let us say, from color A to color B, and vice versa) at a predetermined rate. The experiment showed that for any two colors of the screen, for example A and B, a rate of color change from A to B and from B to A can always be chosen at which the subject sees the color change clearly but does not see the shutter disappearing against the background of the screen. In other words, during a slight change in the apparent color of the screen, the apparent color of the shutter can be changed along with the color of the screen.

With a faster change in the color of the screen, the subject began to observe the shutter. Either disappearing against the background of a relatively unchanged screen or reappearing when the screen was changed, the shutter always appeared as a homogeneous circle to the subject (although it was in fact half black and half white). When the shutter disappeared, the periphery disappeared first, then the center. When it reappeared the effect was sudden, showing the shutter intact, with sharphy defined edges (Fig. 44). When the color of the screen was changed so quickly that the visible color of the shutter could not match the color of the screen, the subject observed that the color change of the shutter clearly lagged behind the color change of the screen. This series of experiments very clearly illustrates the delay mentioned above in seeing the color of the empty field.

If the changes in the screen color reached the rate of 1-3 cycles (illumination changed in a sinusoidal pattern), the apparent color of the shutter could no longer follow the changes in screen color, and the shutter became a uniform hue, a mixture of the changing colors of the screen.

In section 4 of this chapter, we noted that a stationary object (a stationary test field) easily disappears against a background of a flickering environment if the retinal image of this object is illuminated with scattered, flickering light. In the experiments in the present section, the light of a flickering screen, falling on the sclera of the eye, illuminated the whole retina, including the image of the shutter.

In accord with the results described in section 4, it was found that with flicker rates exceeding only 3-6 cycles the differences between the apparent color of the shutter and the screen disappeared, and the area of the visual field corresponding to the shutter appeared to flicker in time with the screen as a whole. It is important to note here that a single cycle or half-cycle of changes in the screen caused appearance on the screen of the shutter which had disappeared, but that a continous series of these cycles caused the shutter to disappear, i.e., caused the screen flicker to spread to the area of the visual field occupied by the shutter. Moreover, the flicker rate at which the shutter disappeared was much lower than the critical rate.

In a series of experiments, a white screen was illuminated by two souces of light. One source threw a constant light on the screen. The illumination color (color A) in this case played no significant part. After an empty field appeared on the shutter (shutter merged with the screen), light flashes of different intensities, spectral composition, and duration were thrown on the screen from the other source. In some experiments the screen illumination was completely switched off for various short time intervals. In all cases, when the duration of the flash or of exclusion of the light did not exceed a few hundredths of a second, the subject observed the shutter only during this interval of time, i.e., while the screen color was distinguishable from the color A, and the apparent color of the shutter, as a result of the delay, remained the same as this color. As soon as the flash ended (if it was not very bright) or the light was switched off the screen resumed color A, and the shutter with its apparent color A again became indistinguishable against its background. The apparent color of the empty field of the shutter began to change appreciably only if the duration of the flash or light exclusion was increased to several tenths of a second. Then, of course, with the end of the flash or of the period of light exclusion, the shutter, having become a different color, remained visible for a short time against the background of the A-color screen.

In the last experiment in section 7 (see description of experiment and Fig. 42), a smooth change was observed from an empty field arising under artificial conditions into an empty field arising under natural conditions. The black-and-white shutter on the screen, which disappeared at the beginning of the experiment, did not subsequently reappear. This fact suggests that the delay in seeing is identical for both empty fields. Differences between these delays would necessarily have revelaed the disappearing shutter when the empty field changed from one state to the other.

Hence, the experiments described in this section have demonstrated the definite delay in seeing the empty field. In a later section, I shall try to show the role of this delay in the process of vision.

9. SPATIAL DEVELOPMENT OF THE FORMATION OF AN EMPTY FIELD

The experiments of section 6 showed that two essentially different processes are part of the work of the visual system—one "fast" and the other "slow." Subsequently the process of perception of contours within the frame of an unchanging and stationary retinal image will be referred to as the "fast" process. This process is assumed to begin at the moment of the last change in the active light, and to end when an empty field forms. To repeat what was said before, it should be noted that the fast process may evidently be associated with the phenomenon, known in electrophysiology, of the appearance of impulses in the optic nerve in response to change in the intensity of light acting on the retina (the on and off effects). The object of the experiments described in this section was to make a more detailed examination of the fast process.

The P_6 cap and adaptors with capillary tubes (described below) were used in these experiments. To anticipate, it may be mentioned that these adaptors can be used to trace the spatial development of the fast process, i.e., they enable the subject to see all stages of this process simultaneously in different experimental conditions.

In many cases in the study of vision it becomes necessary to displace the image of the border between two fields over the retina at a constant and predetermined speed. This purpose can be achieved by means of a capillary tube fixed to the adaptor of the P_6 cap and visible to the subject against the background of the frosted glass reflected in the mirror. One design of such a capillary tube is shown schematically in Fig. 45. The dimensions of the capillary tube, expressed in units of visual angle, are determined from its actual dimensions and the magnification of the short-focus lens.

The internal diameter of the capillary tube is 0.03-0.05 mm. The visual angle subtended by the external diameter of the background C (reflected in the mirror of the frosted glass) is about 45-50°. The bottom part of the capillary tube passes through the center of the background, and its top part is displaced relative to the center by 9-11°. If the axes of symmetry of the cap and the optical system coincide, the lower part of the capillary tube in the field of vision will

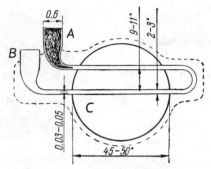

Fig. 45. Diagram of the capillary tube fixed to the adaptor of the P_6 cap (first variant of the adaptor with the capillary tube).

lie at the fovea and the middle of the upper part will cross the region with the highest density of rods. The ends of the capillary tube consist of small curved funnels A and B, the outer diameter of which at their widest part is 0.6 mm. A plug of cotton wool is inserted into one of the funnels but does not project above its edge. The funnels and the parts of the capillary tube projecting outside the adaptor are covered with a layer of glue, shown in Fig. 45 by a broken line; after the glue dries it protects these parts from injury.

An alcoholic solution tinted black with aniline dye is introduced into the funnel A with a micropipet or small brush. The black liquid quickly soaks into the gauze and fills the whole capillary tube. As the liquid evaporates, the meniscus always moves from funnel B to funnel A, i.e., towards the drying pad of compact cotton wool. As the alcohol concentration changes, the intensity of evaporation and the rate of movement of the meniscus of the liquid in the capillary tube also change. The angular velocity of movement of the meniscus visible to the subject through the short-focus lens of the P_6 apparatus can easily be determined, given the length of the capillary tube in degrees and the time taken for the meniscus to move along the capillary tube, measured by the subject with a stopwatch. The velocity of movement of the meniscus in the capillary tube can change from several minutes of angle to several degrees per second. With a slight increase in the evaporation surface of the solution in funnel A, these speeds may be increased 10-20 times. If the inner surface of the capillary tube is clean enough, the meniscus of the colored solution, as it moves along the capillary tubes, leaves no traces; the capillary tube is clean and transparent, and it differs little in color from the frosted glass. During the first second of the experiment the subject sees the meniscus as a sharp, moving boundary between the black liquid and the bright

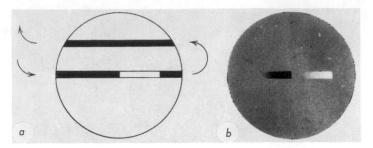

Fig. 46. Scheme to explain the first variant of the adaptor with the capillary tube. a) Image of part of the capillary visible to the subject's eye at the start of the experiment. The black liquid fills the whole capillary tube and moves in the direction indicated by the arrows. In the bottom part of the capillary tube an air bubble can be seen moving together with the fluid; b) subjective appearance of the field a few seconds after the beginning of the experiment, i.e., after the appearance of an empty field.

frosted glass. The background can be colored as desired by covering the beam of light falling on the frosted glass of the cap with colored filters.

As mentioned, the internal diameter of the capillary tube is approximately 0.03-0.05 mm. The mass of liquid in the capillary tube is so small that any sudden movements of the eye in practice will not produce changes in the shape of the meniscus or disturb the smooth, uniform movement of the meniscus in the capillary tube and its image on the retina. If the experiments are carried out at the same temperature with the same solution, the variability of the velocities of movement of the meniscus from one experiment to another will not exceed 5%.

In many experiments it is useful to have two moving menisci at the same time. This can be done as follows. After all the fluid from funnel B has entered the capillary tube, a small volume of solution is inserted into the same funnel from a micropipet, so that a long air bubble is present in the capillary tube between the first and second portions of solution. In this case, two menisci are moving in the subject's field of vision—two boundaries, each of which is a boundary between a white or colored field and a black field. The light is turned on at the anterior boundary of the moving bubble and turned off at the posterior boundary. The subjective appearance of the field in the first moment of the experiment and a few seconds later, i.e., after an empty field has formed, is shown in Fig. 46.

The adaptor by means of which, as in the preceding case, the perception of images moving at a definite speed over the retina can be studied, is illustrated in Fig. 47. The frame of the adaptor 1 is made from black paper glued together. It is a parallelepiped with one edge cut off and covered with paper in which there is a slit. The slit is parallel to the cut-off edge, equal to it in length, and 2.0-2.5 mm wide. Over the slit is glued a thin piece of frosted glass 2, about 0.2 mm in thickness.   Light can enter inside the frame of the adaptor only through the frosted glass. The frosted glass is illuminated with a narrow beam of light so that the sclera of the eye remains in complete darkness.   The bottom part of the adaptor is crossed by capillary tube 3, passing through the axis of symmetry of the cap and parallel to the slit covered by the frosted glass (in Fig. 47 it is perpendicular to the plane of the drawing).

Two small curved funnels 4, joined to both ends of the capillary tube, extend outside the adaptor and are glued to its frame. A small pad of cotton wool soaked in a clear (without coloring matter) solution of alcohol is placed in one funnel.   The internal diameter of the capillary tube and the width of the funnels may be close to the values given in the description of the preceding adaptor, or they may differ from them considerably depending on the experimental condition. At a distance of 1 mm from the capillary tube, a slit 5, slightly wider than the external diameter of the capillary tube, is situated in the base of the adaptor parallel to the capillary tube. The slit is so placed that the eye cannot see the frosted glass. The eye sees only the image of the frosted glass in the capillary tube, magnified by the lens of the P_6 cap. Usually this image appears as a bright band, visible against a completely black background.   The position of the bright band on the segment of the capillary tube filled with liquid and its position on the

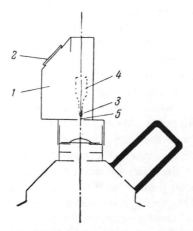

Fig. 47. Second variant of the adaptor with the capillary tube for the P_6 cap.

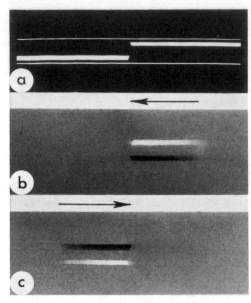

Fig. 48. Scheme to explain the second variant of the adaptor with the capillary tube. a) Capillary tube and meniscus of fluid moving in it, as seen by the subject in the first seconds of the experiment; b) and c) the same capillary tube and meniscus as seen by the subject after the appearance of an empty field. The arrows indicate the direction of movement of the meniscus.

segment free from liquid are displaced approximately as shown in Fig. 48a. In this case, movement of the meniscus in the capillary tube takes the form of movement of two boundaries. Movement of one boundary is accompanied by turning the light on, movement of the other by turning it off. The subjective appearance of the field after the formation of an empty field is shown in Fig. 48b and c. The width, the number, and the position of the images of the frosted glass in the capillary tube are determined by the relative positions of the frosted glass and capillary tube, and are predetermined by the experimenter as he makes the adaptor. In some cases, it is desirable to use a capillary tube oval, not round, in cross section. Sometimes, to simplify the field as it appears to the subject, the width of the slit 5 is reduced and part of the capillary tube is covered, leaving only the brightest band. The angular velocities of movement of the meniscus are determined and regulated just as in the first variant of the adaptor with the capillary tube. Depending on the purpose of the experiment, the experimenter may use the first or second variant of the adaptor. With the first variant, nearly the whole retina is illuminated with the bright background of the frosted glass, while in the second nearly all the retina is in darkness.

After the cap had been applied to the eye and an empty field had appeared, depending on the construction of the adaptor, the field appeared to the subject as illustrated in Fig. 46 or 48. As he vividly expressed it, the subject saw apparently "two comets," moving over the background of an empty field. One of the comets appeared bright and the other very black ("much blacker than the dark background of the empty field"). Later we shall describe the bright comet conventionally as the on-comet and the dark as the off-comet (since the first corresponds to the turned-on light, the second to the turned-off light). If the fast process can be associated with the on and off effects, the spatial evolution of the fast process may be regarded as analogous to the trains of impulses in the optic nerve.

The anterior part of each comet contained an area of uniform color. The apparent color of these areas then changed smoothly into that of the empty field.

To determine the time characteristics of the fast process, the apparent length of the comets was measured. During the experiments, a shadow from a narrow strip of paper was thrown onto the frosted glass. Since the shadow moved across the frosted glass, it could be seen, although not very sharply, by the subject against the background of the empty field. When the shadow was near the comet, the subject compared the width of the shadow and the length of the comet. It was always possible to choose a strip of paper giving a shadow of width equal to the length of the comet. After the experiment, the width of the shadow in units of visual angle was measured. Since the angular velocity of the comet was known, all the information required to give the time characteristics of the fast process was available.

The border between two fields moving over the background of an empty field produces a sharp change in the illuminance of a certain part of the retina and, consequently, leads to the appearance of the fast process. Since the boundary moves at a constant speed over the retina, conditions are produced in which the subject can observe all stages of the fast process at the same time.

The next step was an attempt to discover how the application of certain stimuli affects the apparent length and color of the comet in conditions when these stimuli involve only part of the retina. Against the background of an empty field, and very close to the on- and off-comets, objects of different color and luminance, with an angular diameter of about 5-7°, moved and therefore were visible. No appreciable change was observed in the length and color of the comets.

When these objects coincided with the comets, the color of the comets appeared to change only in the segments immediately next to the moving object.

If part of the capillary tube was shaded with transverse black bands, the subject saw the comet broken up into isolated segments when it passed through this area. These conditions did not appear to alter the total length and color of the on- and off-comets. With the accuracy attainable with this method, it was found that the length of the comets changed proportionally to the speed of movement of the menisci.

In face of these results, the comets may be regarded as the evolution of the fast process in space. In fact, if the action of the stimuli on the areas of the retina lying next to the comet in the visual field had not influenced its apparent length and color, evidently the action of the meniscus image could not have influenced the areas through which it had already passed and which corresponded to the extinction of the fast process. In addition, it was found that the duration of the fast process, measured by the time required for appearance of the empty field, and the duration of the fast process, measured by means of the comets, coincided approximately (I say "approximately" because the subject found it difficult to determine the moment when all contours disappeared from the test field).

When movement of the image over the retina was fairly slow, the menisci could not be seen, and consequently no comets appeared. For instance, when a bright light fell on the sclera and the luminance of the frosted glass of the cap was 500 apostilbs, if the meniscus moved with a velocity relative to the retina of 18-19 minutes of angle per second, the subject could see nothing, but if the speed was 23-24 minutes of angle per second, the subject could see the on- and off-comets. If the experiments were carried out without illumination of the sclera, through which scattered light usually falls on the retina, appearance of the comets was observed by the subject when the meniscus moved at a speed of 3-5 minutes of angle per second.

As mentioned above, the first part of each comet had an area of uniform color, which then appeared to change gradually into the color of the empty field. Evidently the presence of this area indicates that the fast process in its initial stage shows little variation, and that extinction begins only after a short time. The duration of the initial, relatively constant part of the fast process was approximately 1-3 sec; extinction of this process took 2-5 sec.

A change in the spectral composition of the light falling on the frosted glass of the cap caused no change in the apparent length of the comets. The on-comet always took the color of the frosted glass, while the off-comet appeared black, tinged with a color complementary to the color of the on-comet. If the intensity of the light falling on the frosted glass was increased by two or three orders, there was a slight increase in the apparent length of the comets.

An attempt was then made to examine the behavior of the comets when the illuminance of the eye was sharply varied. When the cornea is covered by the cap, it is easy to change the illuminance of the whole retina with scattered light by changing the intensity of illumination of the sclera. A sudden change in illuminance may cause the comets to contract or completely disappear. It was always possible to change the luminance of the retina in such a way that objects disappearing for the subject because of the immobility of the retinal image hardly appeared at all, while changes in the comets under these conditions were clearly apparent to the subject.

I simply wish to emphasize here the fact that a change in illuminance leads, in particular, to the complete or partial inhibition of the fast process (the comet contracts or disappears for an instant, then recovers). This phenomenon is evidently analogous to the process of pre-excitatory inhibition, familiar in the electrophysiology of the retina. Pre-excitatory inhibition is clearly seen on records of impulses obtained from the optic nerve of animals. An example of this inhibition, in the optic nerve of a frog, is shown in Fig. 49.

The P_7 cap was used (see the description of this apparatus) to examine the behavior of the fast processes in conditions close to the usual conditions of perception. The stationary test field was a capillary tube similar to the capillary tube from the first type of adaptor (Fig. 45). When the cap was in position, the image of the surrounding objects and the image of the capillary tube were superimposed on each other on the retina. For the first few seconds, the subject saw a sharp image of the capillary tube as a shadow superimposed on the object used for fixation. Then, since the capillary tube was immobile relative to the retina, the shadow disappeared and reappeared slightly only if change in the points of fixation was accompanied by a considerable change in the color of the background object. When the capillary tube was no longer seen by the subject, the movement of the meniscus of the black liquid inside the capillary tube evoked the appearance of on- and off-comets. The subject saw the comets against the background of the surrounding object; the faint image of the capillary tube that sometimes appeared during change in the points of fixation did not prevent him from making observations on the comets.

The following experiment was carried out. Three screens were placed before the subject. One was cardboard checkered with pieces

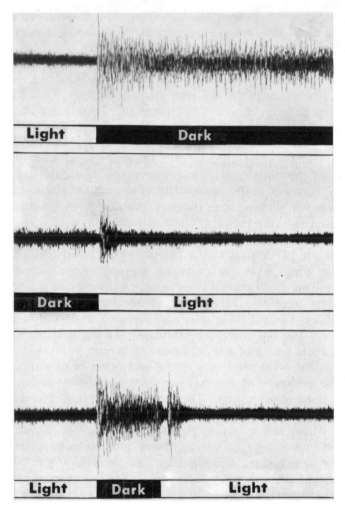

Fig. 49. Records of optic-nerve impulses of the frog (*Rana ridibunda*). Impulses appearing in response to the change from light to dark and from dark to light are shown in the bottom photograph. During the change from dark to light, the impulses continue at first, but then are completely inhibited. This pre-excitatory inhibition is clearly seen on the records.

of paper of different colors glued to it. The two halves of the second screen differed very slightly in color. The third screen was a sheet of paper of uniform color and intensity of illumination. The subject saw each screen at such an angle that the image of the capillary tube, and consequently the comet, was superimposed on its background.

During the experiment the subject examined the screens in turn and adjusted the points of fixation so that the comets did not go outside the boundaries of the screen. When the subject changed the points of fixation on the first (checkered) screen, each such change was accompanied by a momentary disappearance of the on- and off-comets, which then reappeared because of the movement of the head of the comet. When the subject adjusted the points of fixation on the second screen so that at the moment the change was made the background on which the comets were seen was slightly changed, the comets contracted, then returned to their original size. Adjustment of the points of fixation on the third (solid-color) screen did not visibly alter the length of the on- and off-comets.

It may be assumed that the contraction and disappearance of the comets described above should be regarded as indications of the complete or partial inhibition of the fast process, corresponding to those parts of the retina on which the changes in the comets were seen at the moment of, and after, the change in the points of fixation. The experiments described above confirm that, depending on changes in illuminance taking place as a result of a change in points of fixation, the fast processes on various parts of the retina may be completely inhibited, partly inhibited, or not inhibited at all.

During fixation on an object, the human eye is constantly in movement, making small but rapid rotations. These eye movements are accompanied by the appearance and inhibition of a series of fast processes, corresponding to those parts of the retina over which the image of sharply defined elements of the object moves as a result of the eye movements. The apparent color of the empty field situated inside an object of uniform color is determined by its surroundings; the visual system extrapolates to the empty field the color visible at the edges of the surface. What we extrapolate with is discrete (alternation of fast processes and inhibitions as a result of saccadic eye movements), and what we obtain by extrapolation is continuous (the apparent color of the empty field is unchanged during the time that the observer fixates on the object). However, this is understandable in view of the existence of a delay in seeing the color of the empty field. This delay enables us, when extrapolating from the edges of a uniform surface, to see it unchanged in color when the image of the borders moves continually and saccadically over the retina, which in turn is essential to enable us to see these borders.

At this point it should be noted that each sudden rotation of the eyes during fixation lasts about 0.02 sec, and the duration does not exceed 3% of the total fixation time. During the sharp change in the environment of the empty field, appreciable changes in its apparent color take place only after a delay of several tenths of a second.

10. PERCEPTION OF OBJECTS MOVING
ON AN EMPTY FIELD

I have previously described experiments in which objects moved across an empty field. Let us now consider this case in rather more detail. To facilitate the description, I shall use the word "objects" to describe test fields mobile relative to the retina, moving against the background of an empty field.

In the first series of experiments in this section the P_6 cap was used, and the color of the stationary test field varied widely from experiment to experiment. In each experiment, after the appearance of an empty field, a black object 3° in diameter was moved across it. This caused no change in the apparent color of the empty field, but sometimes a small halo appeared around the moving object. It may be supposed that these haloes appeared as a result of extrapolations similar to those discussed in section 7. In this case, however, the extrapolation was directed inward, and not outward, from the border of the moving surface. The essential feature so far as we are concerned is that no differences in the stationary test field appeared inside the halo. The apparent color of the black object coincided with the color of the after-image arising when the light was completely switched off. This can be understood because the appearance of a black object in the field of vision and the exclusion of light falling on this part of the retina are in practice identical processes. It was then found that the apparent color of the black object depends not only on the color of the stationary test field, but also on the speed of movement of the object. This is because the color of the after-image changes in time, and, depending on the character of the movements of the object, the appearance and disappearance of the after-image will differ.

At this point it is well to recall the experiments discussed in a previous section. In these experiments, a bright white object moved against the background of an empty field. The diameter of the object was 3°. Its luminance in all the experiments was much greater than that of the stationary test field. These experiments showed that the color of the empty field appeared unchanged, while the white object at first (immediately after the appearance of the empty field) appeared white, but changed appreciably during the next 30-40 sec, eventually acquiring a saturated hue approximately complementary to the color of the stationary test field.

In one experiment in which the P_6 cap was used, the stationary test field was a bright white field—the frosted glass of the cap (Fig. 50).

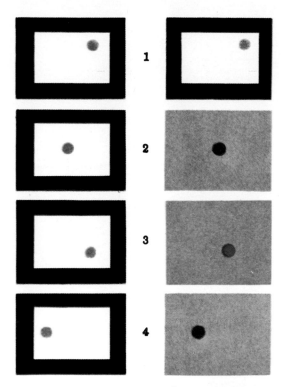

Fig. 50. Scheme of an experiment. In each pair of figures, the stationary test field and the red object moving against its background (the mobile test field) are shown on the left. The right-hand figure of each pair shows the appearance of the test field and object in different experimental conditions. 1) Test field and its apparent color at the beginning of the experiment; 2) after 1-3 sec an empty field formed and the color of the object appeared to change; 3) when the second eye was illuminated with red light, the color of the empty field and of the object appeared to change; 4) when the second eye was illuminated with blue light the next moment, color of the empty field and object again appeared to change.

Fig. 51. Scheme of an experiment. In each pair of figures, the red screen (mobile test field) and the black-and-white shutter (stationary test field) placed against it are shown on the left. The right figure in each pair shows the appearance of the test field. 1) Test field and its apparent color at the beginning of the experiment; 2) after 1-3 sec an empty field formed on the shutter, and its color appeared to merge with the color of the screen. Next the experimenter moved a red circle in front of the white half of the shutter. The actual color of the circle coincided with that of the screen. The subject saw only a moving circle whose color appeared darker and more saturated than the color of the screen; 3) when the experimenter then moved the circle in front of the black half of the shutter, the moving circle appeared to the subject to be less saturated in color and much lighter than the screen.

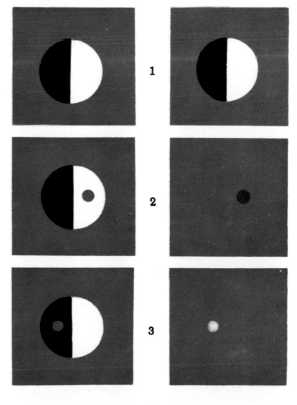

Against the background of this field moved a red object, 3° in diameter, the luminance of which was much less than the luminance of this field. The experiments showed that with the appearance of the empty field, when the color of the white test field had appeared to become dark gray, the color of the red object appeared to change from red to dark red and then remained appreciably darker than the empty field. Later the subject's second eye was illuminated with red light, as a result of which the color of the empty field appeared to become red, and the color of the object appeared more saturated; the object was now "very red," and as before, appreciably darker than the empty field. When the subject's second eye was illuminated with blue light, the color of the empty field acquired a blue tinge, and the color of the red object appeared to lose much of its saturation, becoming dark brown, and as in all the previous cases, remaining much darker than the empty field.

Although the color of the background on which the object moved and the color of the object itself appeared to change sharply with the change in the experimental conditions, the character of the difference existing between the stationary test field and the object was the same at all stages of the experiment.

The result of one experiment in which the P_8 cap was used is illustrated in Fig. 51. In this experiment, the mobile test field was a large, well-lighted sheet of red paper, on which was placed the stationary test field (the shutter), half black and half white. The diameter of the stationary test field was 20°. The movable object was a small red circle, the same color as the mobile test field and 3° in diameter. The question was: what was the apparent color of the object moved against the empty field arising on the shutter? Not only was the real color of the red object equal to that of the mobile test field, but the apparent color of the empty field in these experimental conditions also became equal to the color of this same mobile test field.

The subject could clearly see the object moving against the background of the empty field, although he could not see the empty field itself. When against the right half of the empty field, the object appeared to the subject to be an extremely saturated red color, darker than the mobile test field. When on the left half of the empty field, the object appeared pink, lighter than the mobile test field. Sometimes small haloes were observed around the object. Here, as in the previous experiment, a tendency was observed for the character of the differences between the stationary test field and the object (in brightness and color) to persist.

11. ROLE OF ILLUMINATION OF THE EYE WITH SCATTERED LIGHT

Experimenters investigating human vision do not usually attach great importance to light falling on the retina through the sclera. This is natural, because with more or less constant intensity of illumination (and consequently constant illuminance) scattered light falling on the retina has little effect on the results of many experiments. However, when working with stabilized images, it is particularly important to exclude light or to make it as constant as possible, because (see section 5) any suprathreshold decrease in illuminance reveals contours in a test field that have disappeared because of immobility (with any suprathreshold addition of illuminance the subject sees only this addition). In most cases a significant change in illuminance may be produced not only by accidental changes in the intensity of illumination, but also by rotation of the eye or by a shadow flickering on the sclera.

Let us first consider the phenomena arising in conditions of flickering illuminance of great brightness. In one of the experiments with the P_3 cap, the cornea was completely covered, and light could enter the eye only through the sclera. The eyelids were retracted as widely as possible with strips of adhesive plaster and a bright flickering light was thrown onto the sclera. Usually, with a flicker frequency of 6 to 15 cycles, the subject saw bright mosaics, iridescent with all the colors of the rainbow. These mosaics had very saturated colors; they were small in the region of the fovea and larger at the periphery of the retina. The picture was particularly colorful at the times that the flicker frequency was raised or lowered.

Next, the P_6 cap was placed on the subject's eye, allowing scattered light to pass into the eye only through the cornea and pupil, i.e., only through the transparent media of the eye (illumination through the sclera was excluded). In this case, the bright colors of the mosaic which had appeared immediately faded, although its faint tints were still perceptible. However, as soon as an orange filter (Schott OG-2) was introduced into the beam of light falling on the frosted glass of the cap the mosaic again acquired the same bright and varied colors.

These experiments reveal the role of illumination of the retina by flickering light through the sclera, which behaves like the orange filter. These results also demonstrate the care required in interpreting results of experiments in which a fluctuating light falls on the sclera. The actual hue of light entering the eye through the sclera can easily be determined as follows. In a completely dark room the temporal part of a subject's sclera is illuminated with a bright beam of light. Under these conditions, as the experimenter will see, the whole inner region of the eye shines with an orange light. This experiment clearly shows the background of illumination against which a retinal image is formed when the sclera is brightly illuminated.

In a series of experiments the illumination of the retina with flickering light was carried out both through the sclera and through the frosted glass of the cap. Sometimes these two forms of illumination were synchronized for the frosted glass and sclera; sometimes they were not. In some experiments the illumination of different parts of the sclera and that of different parts of the frosted glass were out of phase. In these experiments the subject often saw geometrical figures, fantastic in their complexity, variety, and color, with their center in the foveal part of the retina. Although much space could be devoted to the description of these experiments we would be no nearer to understanding these phenomena. I can only suggest that the complex, unusual changes of a bright color on the retina lead to confusion of information at certain levels of the visual system, as a result of which the subject sees these remarkable visual phenomena. The experiments of this series were a severe strain on some subjects. Subjects for such experiments should be chosen with particular care.

I next tried to discover how much the color appearance of the test field depends on the fact that the optic fundus is colored orange by pigments and blood vessels. In these experiments the test field, stationary relative to the retina, was illuminated with white light of varying intensity. Light reached the retina only through the transparent media of the eye.

The experiments showed that the white test field, having disappeared because of its immobility, in the presence of a gradual and suprathreshold increase in the luminance of the white screen, caused a sensation of yellow. A gradual suprathreshold decrease in the luminance of the white test field lent an appreciably bluish color to this field. If the disappearing test field were bright enough, the blue color that developed would appear saturated to the subject.

It is possible that the results obtained were due to the orange color of the optic fundus and so must be taken into consideration in experiments with a test field of variable intensity (or color).

To determine how the eye adapts itself to certain anomalies in illumination, stationary relative to the retina, several experiments were carried out using the P_7 and P_8 caps. By means of the P_7 cap, dark shadows (stationary relative to the retina) were formed on different parts of the retina. When the shadows were superimposed on the retinal image in the process of perception, each shadow, roughly speaking, uniformly cut off a certain constant fraction of the light. Instead of a shutter, different neutral and colored filters were fixed to the P_8 cap. By means of the neutral filter, the illuminance of the retinal image could be reduced by a specified number of times on a particular part of the retina.

These experiments showed that within a few seconds the subject ceased to notice the presence of even dark shadows and filters (absorbing, for example, 70-90% of the light) if he looked at uniform surfaces or at objects with details possessing slight contrast of light and color. If the subject examined very checkered or contrasty surfaces, the shadows and filters could still be noticed to some extent. Faint shadows and weak filters (absorbing, for example, 20-30% of the light) were practically unnoticed by the subject even against a checkered background.

These experiments suggest that although the human eye is well adapted to certain constant and stationary anomalies in illumination of the retina, it cannot become completely adapted to them (at least in the course of one single experiment).

CONCLUSIONS

We may draw the following conclusions from the results of the experiments described in Chapter II. For optimal working conditions of the human visual system, some degree of constant (interrupted or uninterrupted) movement of the retinal image is essential. If a test field (of any size, color, and luminance) becomes and remains strictly constant and stationary relative to the retina, it will become and remain an empty field within 1-3 sec.

Very often, conditions of steady illumination arise on certain parts of the retina in the process of perception. Such conditions arise during the perception of large and uniform surfaces and during small movements of the eyes. If the illumination continues constant for more than three seconds, an empty field appears inside this uniform surface (or surfaces). The empty field always takes the color of the surroundings and, in ordinary conditions, is never seen by the human subject. In other words, the visual system extrapolates the apparent color of the edges of the surface to its center. In accordance with electrophysiological findings, I suggest that in man constancy and immobility of the retinal image will banish impulses entering the optic nerve from the eye or will sharply reduce their number. In these circumstances, absence of signals from a certain part of the retina gives the visual system information that this area corresponds to a uniform surface, the color of which does not change and is equal to the color of its edges.

It may be concluded that the visual system "identifies" the empty field arising in artificial conditions with the empty field arising in natural conditions. For this reason, the empty field arising in artificial conditions always appears to the subject as a uniform background (all visible contours disappear inside the field), and the apparent color of the field is always the color of its surroundings.

Two essentially different processes are found in the work of the visual system: the first, a fast process of disappearance of all contours in a stationary test field; the second, a slow process which usually is easily detected by means of after-images. The fast process may evidently be associated with the appearance of impulses in the optic nerve in response to a change in the intensity of light (the on- and off-effects familiar from electrophysiology). The second, slow process is evidently associated with a change in the state of the retina—with its adaptation.

A definite delay is found in seeing the color of an empty field. This delay enables us, by extrapolating from the edges of a uniform surface, to see this surface unchanged in color when the image of the edges is continuously and saccadically displaced over the retina; this in turn is essential in order that we can see these edges.

Chapter III

EYE MOVEMENTS DURING FIXATION
ON STATIONARY OBJECTS

Before describing the material contained in this chapter, I shall try to explain the general character of eye movements during the perception of stationary objects. Let us consider Fig. 52, which shows a recording of the movements of a subject's two eyes when examining a flat picture with one eye. During the experiment one of the subject's eyes was covered by a P_2 cap and the other with a P_1 cap. The black dots in Fig. 52 show the points of fixation during perception of the picture, and the thin lines show movement of each eye from point to point. During the recording, the picture was in a frontal plane. In this case, change in the points of fixation was, roughly speaking, accomplished by movements of a single type—identical and simultaneous very rapid rotation of the eyes, hereinafter conventionally termed "saccades."

At this point, I should stress that in any situation, the saccades of the eyes are of high velocity (the duration of a saccade is measured in hundredths of a second) and uniform amplitude, and both eyes move simultaneously. It is clear from Fig. 52 that this last property is preserved even when one eye is completely covered by a cap, i.e., is excluded from perception.

Some readers may think that during the perception of stationary objects the human eyes are able to perform smooth pursuing movements in addition to saccades. Where stationary objects are concerned, this view is incorrect. It is due to the fact that the small saccades of the eyes are performed involuntarily and we are not aware of them. A record of eye movements is shown in Fig. 53, during which the subject tried to follow the lines of several geometrical figures with his eyes smoothly (without saccades). Although subjectively the tracking movements of the eyes seemed smooth and uninterrupted, they were in fact,

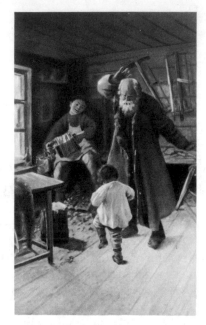

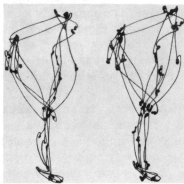

Fig. 52. A reproduction of A.L. Rzhevskaya's picture "A Happy Minute" with records of the movement of each eye during free (without instruction) examination of the reproduction by one eye for a period of 30 sec (the second eye was completely covered by a P_2 cap).

as the record shows, composed of discrete stops and small saccades. Again in Fig. 53, we can see that the involuntary saccades arising during the attempt to trace the lines of the figures visually did not invariably lie along these lines.

   If the observer carefully examines any point of a stationary object, he imagines objectively that he is fixating on this point with motionless eyes.   Records show that in fact this process is accompanied by involuntary saccades of which the observer is unaware (sometimes resembling spasms of the eyes). The experiment showed that it is not only the small saccades (measuring from 2 to 20 minutes of angle) which are involuntary. Large saccades (usually not exceeding 15-20°) also are mainly involuntary, and the observer is not aware of them during perception.

When the object of perception is stationary relative to the observer's head, the process of perception taking place between any two adjacent saccades in the following pages will be conventionally called "fixation process." It has been shown experimentally that during the perception of stationary objects, in the interval between rotations of

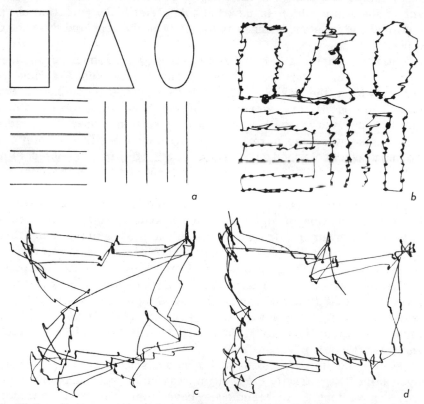

Fig. 53. Record of eye movements during examination of geometrical figures. a) Geometrical figures presented to the subject for examination; b) record of eye movements during which the subject tried to trace the lines of the figures with his eye smoothly and without saccades; c) record of eye movements during free (without instruction) examination of the figures for 20 sec; d) record of eye movements during examination of the figures for 20 sec after the instruction "look at the figures and count the number of straight lines."

the head and blinking movements, the human eyes can be only in one of two states: in a state of fixation or in a state of changing the points of fixation. The present chapter is devoted to the study of eye movements during fixation directed to any element of a stationary object. Accordingly, we shall examine the fixation process and the small involuntary saccades of the eyes.

It follows from the facts described in Chapter II that slight movement of the eyes is essential for good conditions of perception, even in the case of fixation on the elements of stationary objects. Fixation, recorded in Figs. 52 and 53 as black dots, is accompanied by two or three types of movements: drifts, tremor, and involuntary saccades. In addition, we must always remember that some displacement of the retinal image and change in the image itself may be caused by movement of the head, which is never absolutely still, by pulsation of the blood, and by constant changes in the state of the lens and the size of the pupil.

A drift is an irregular and relatively slow movement of the axes of the eyes, in which the image of the fixation point for each eye remains within the fovea. The drift is always accompanied by a tremor, an oscillatory movement of the axes of the eyes of high frequency but very small amplitude. Small involuntary saccades usually arise when the duration of fixation on a particular point of a stationary object exceeds a certain length of time (0.3-0.5 sec) or when, because of drifts, the image of the point of fixation becomes too far removed from the center of the fovea. Not all fixations are accompanied by involuntary saccades. For instance, during a relatively cursory examination of an object, most fixations are accompanied by two types of movement, drift and tremor. The most suitable conditions for recording drift, tremor, and involuntary saccadic movements of the eyes occur during prolonged fixation on a stationary point.

The general (saccadic) character of the eye movements has been known for a long time and has been studied by many authors (Müller, 1826; Lamansky, 1869; Javal, 1879; Landolt, 1891; Delabarre, 1898; Orschansky, 1899; Huey, 1898, 1900; Judd, McAllister, and Steele, 1905; Dodge, 1907; others).

Despite the imperfections of the methods used by these authors, they obtained a generally correct impression of the fundamental type of eye movement. As techniques have improved, more and more investigations of eye movements have been made. Attention has been directed in particular to the fixation process, in which the role of eye movements in all its details was not clear. Very often the same problems were studied by many investigators using different methods.

I shall not mention all these investigations, some of which duplicated each other. My purpose is to show, using the best method available, how micromovements of the eyes prevent the formation of an empty field in the fixation process.

1. DRIFT OF THE OPTICAL AXES DURING FIXATION

The drift of the axes of the eyes was first discovered, and on the whole correctly described, by Dodge (1907). He considered that there is no constant point of fixation and suggested the term "fixation field." Subsequently, nearly all authors studying eye movements confirmed the presence of drifting movements of the eyes (Glezer and Tsukkerman, 1961). An exception in this case was Hartridge (1947) in whose opinion fixation can take place with an accuracy of up to one cone unit.

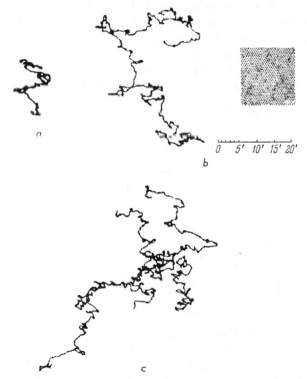

Fig. 54. Records of eye movements during fixation on a stationary point by the subject. a) Fixation for 10 sec; b) fixation for 30 sec; c) fixation for 1 min. The scale of angular measurement in minutes of angle is given in record b, and the distribution of the cones is indicated schematically on this scale.

It is clear from Figs. 52 and 53 that fixations accompanying the perception of images are recorded not as points, but as irregularly shaped spots. The size and shape of these spots are determined by the drift of the optical axes of the eyes. To obtain a general idea of drifts, let us first examine Fig. 54, in which the spots produced by drifts are greatly magnified. This figure consists of three separate recordings of eye movements (with exposures of 10, 30, and 60 seconds) made on stationary photosensitive paper by means of the P_1 cap. Each record shows only the drifts of the eye during fixation. In the same figure, a small area of the retina (the fovea) is shown on a corresponding scale. The records given in Fig. 54 (and others like them) show that the drift of the eye axis during fixation is an irregular movement during which, however, the image of the point of fixation always remains inside the fovea. There are two reasons for this: first, there is a definite constancy in fixation of the angle between the optical axes of the eyes (the angle of convergence) and second, involuntary correcting saccades of the eyes occur, returning the image of the points closer to the center of the fovea. Analysis of these records shows that the drift speed varied chaotically from zero to approximately 30 minutes of angle per second. During fixation, purely as a result of drift, the axis of the eye moves with a mean velocity of approximately 6 minutes

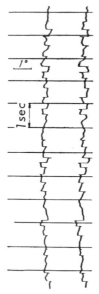

Fig. 55. Horizontal component of the movements of the two eyes on a photokymograph during fixation by the subject on a stationary point.

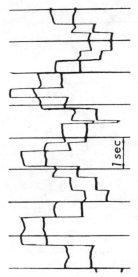

Fig. 56. Horizontal component of the movements of the two eyes on a photokymograph during examination by the subject of a stationary picture.

of angle per second and, consequently, moves in one second along a path equal to 10–15 diameters of the cones of the central part of the fovea. It is very significant that, as a rule, several times per second for periods measured in hundredths and tenths of a second, the drift reaches almost maximal values, i.e., about 30 minutes of angle per second (speeds at which no empty field can develop). Ditchburn recently (1959) obtained a mean value of the speed of drift of 5 minutes of angle per second.

Let us now turn to Figs. 55 and 56. Figure 55 is a record of the horizontal component of the movements of both eyes during fixation on a stationary point. The record was made on the vertically moving tape of a slit photokymograph by means of a P_1 cap. It is clear from this figure that the saccades of both eyes were always equal, whereas the drift was largely independent for each eye (the vertical lines do not remain parallel. The scales of Figs. 55 and 56 precluded recording of tremor.

Figure 56 (like Fig. 55) is also a record of the horizontal component of the movements of both eyes, but during free and cursory examination of a stationary object (in this case, the nature of the object does not matter). The records in Fig. 56 resemble those of Fig. 55 in many respects. However, the saccades of the eyes recorded in Fig. 56 are changes in the points of fixation and each individual act of fixation is accompanied only by drift and tremor. It is clear from Fig. 56 that

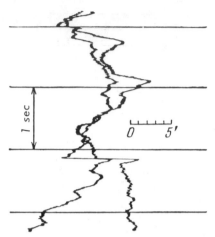

Fig. 57. Horizontal component of the movements of the two eyes recorded on a photo-kymograph during fixation by the subject on a stationary point. This record clearly shows that the drifts and the tremor shown by one eye are independent of those shown by the other eye.

during free examination of a stationary object the drift of each eye is independent of the other. Finally, in Fig. 57 the independence of and difference between the drifts of the two eyes are recorded on a scale at which the tremor is perceptible. The drift lying between two successive saccades will conventionally be called an independent drift.

Many records have shown that during the free examination of stationary objects, the overwhelming majority of fixations on elements of the object take place without saccades (involuntary). For such fixations the duration of the independent drifts and the duration of fixation are identical. It is important during perception of a stationary object that the duration of the independent drift (of fixation) is nearly always adequate to enable the eye to see the fixated element. However, this time may sometimes be insufficient for the thought process evoked by the perceived element to be completed. Usually, our gaze is directed towards the element about which we think; in which case, a prolonged fixation arises, composed of independent drifts and involuntary saccades. It may be concluded that the same element is seen repeatedly during such a fixation, although the observer usually is unaware of the brief interruptions caused by the involuntary saccades.

A graph of the distribution of the independent drifts of the eye in accordance with their duration during the free examination of a picture, i.e., a graph of the distribution of fixations in accordance with their duration, is given in Fig. 58. The P_1 cap was used in these experi-

ments.   The record was made on a photokymograph on which the tape
moved at a speed of 20 cm/sec, and the time marker showed each
0.2 sec.   In this way an accuracy of measurement of ±0.005 sec was
obtained.   A device mounted on the photokymograph allowed simultaneous recording of the horizontal and vertical movements of the eyes.

It may be concluded from this graph that during free examination
of stationary objects the most probable duration of the drifts (fixations)
was from 0.3 to 0.8 sec.   In particular, the marked increase on the
graph in the number of drifts when their duration was over 0.20 sec
should be noted. This suggests that for optimal perception of stationary

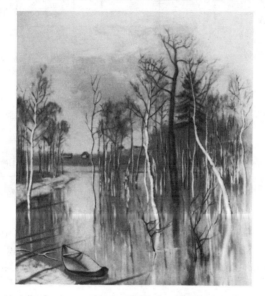

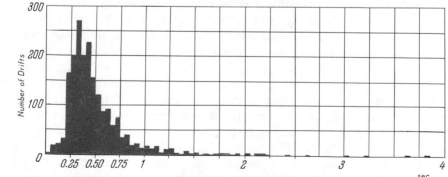

Fig. 58. Reproduction of I.I. Levitan's picture "The Flood" shown to five observers for free
examination, and graph of the distribution of 2000 drifts in accordance with their duration.
Abscissas—duration of the drifts; ordinate—number of drifts of approximately equal duration.

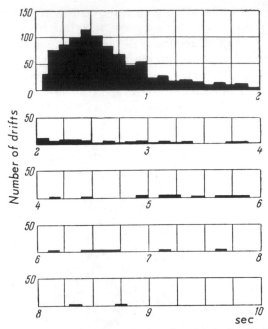

Fig. 59. Distribution of 1000 drifts in relation to their duration during fixation on a stationary point. The results for four observers are given. Abscissa—duration of the drifts; ordinate—number of drifts of approximately equal duration.

objects, the lower limit of duration of the fixations should be taken as 0.25 sec. The graph also shows that, in the conditions described, the duration of the drift (fixation) most commonly found was 0.3 sec.

The mean duration of eye drift is to some extent dependent on the subject and his state, on the character of the visual test object, and on the instruction which the subject receives before the experiment. For example, during continuous and prolonged fixation on a point, when the subject has been told to fixate on it continuously, the distribution of independent drifts in relation to their duration (Fig. 59) differs appreciably from the picture seen in Fig. 58. The duration of the independent drifts is noticeably greater, sometimes amounting to several seconds. In certain diseases, the drifts show a definite direction instead of being irregular (sometimes in healthy observers also). In this case, of course, a drift taking place predominantly towards one side is corrected by small saccades in the opposite direction. This fact has been recorded in healthy subjects by Nachmias (1959).

Experiments have shown that when an observer tries to fixate on a point for a long time about 97% of the time is given over to drifts and only 3% to saccades. During free examination of a flat, stationary picture, depending on the size and character of the picture, saccades may account for more than 3-5% of the time. Finally, when the free perception of a stationary object is accompanied by a change in the points of the fixation in space, so that convergence and divergence of the eyes take place, considerably more than 5% of the total perception time may be taken up in changing the points of fixation.

2. TREMOR OF THE EYES

Of all forms of eye movements, tremor is the most difficult to study. The amplitude of the tremor is very low and its frequency very high; this complicates recording of the tremor because movement of the subject's head, as well as the vibration of the apparatus and of the building itself, must be taken into account during recording. In addition, the recording of tremor imposes serious demands on the optical system used in the investigation. The first records of tremor were made by Adler and Fliegelman (1934); later records were made by Ratliff and Riggs (1950, 1951) and Ditchburn and Ginsborg (1953).

My own records of tremor date from 1956. Other authors also have frequently recorded tremor. Most records have shown that the amplitude of the tremor (its angular dimensions) is comparable with the angular dimensions of the eye receptors, while its frequency varies

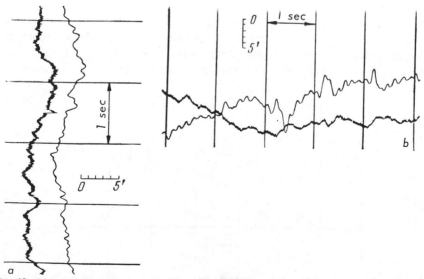

Fig. 60. Photokymographic records of movements of the eye and an upper incisor tooth of a subject during fixation on a stationary point. a) Horizontal component; b) vertical of records.

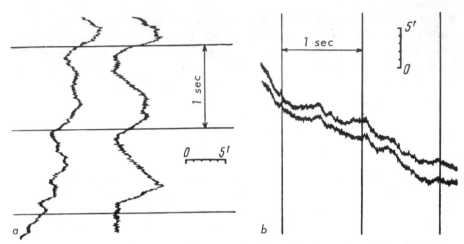

Fig. 61. Photokymographic record of movements of the subject's two eyes during fixation on a stationary point. a) Horizontal component; b) vertical component of the record.

from 30 to 90 cycles. Ditchburn (1959) notes that tremor is characterized by a continuous spectrum of frequencies up to 150 cps.

As mentioned earlier, any drift of the eyes is accompanied by tremor, but the two forms of movement are independent. To obtain a general idea of tremor, let us consider Figs. 60 and 61. These figures show records of the horizontal and vertical components of the eye movements on a scale at which the tremor can be seen. The records were made on the moving tape of a photokymograph by means of the P_1 cap. Parallel and simultaneous records of the eye movements and the movements of an upper tooth (an incisor, to which a small mirror was attached during the experiment), to differentiate between the

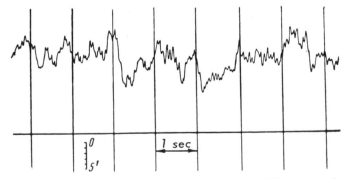

Fig. 62. Photokymographic record of the horizontal component of the tremor of a stationary hand resting on the table, and of the vibration of the chin rest (straight line).

movements of the eye and the movements of the head, are shown in Fig. 60. It is clear from this figure that the high frequencies characteristic of the tremor of the eyes were not recorded with the head movements.

Parallel and simultaneous records of the eye movements are shown in Fig. 61. For comparison the tremor of hand and the vibration of chin rest (Fig. 62) were recorded under the same conditions. In these experiments, the chin rest was fixed to a massive frame mounted on a felt cushion. During the experiment illustrated in Fig. 62, the subject's hand rested on the chin rest. Recordings such as those in Figs. 60, 61, and 62 show convincingly that the high-frequency oscillations recorded on the photokymograph tapes are not an artifact but correspond to the eye movements customarily called tremor.

Analysis of the records I obtained of tremor yielded the following results. The amplitude of the tremor is 20–40 seconds of angle (1.0–1.5 diameter of the cones in the fovea). The tremor is composed mainly of movements whose frequency is 70–90 oscillations per second (much higher than the critical frequency of flicker fusion). As a result of tremor, the axis of the eye moves over a conical surface, covering each such surface in approximately 0.011–0.013 sec. In other words, if the axis of the eye is mentally continued to its intersection with the frontal plane, as a result of the tremor it will describe elliptical figures on that plane.

3. SMALL INVOLUNTARY SACCADES OF THE EYES

It is relatively simple to record saccades, and many investigators have long held the correct view that saccades for both eyes coincide in time, in amplitude, and in direction. The small involuntary saccades of the eyes were first discovered by Dodge (1907).

To examine in rather more detail the small involuntary saccades arising during prolonged fixation on a stationary point, let us turn to Fig. 63. This graph shows the distribution of small involuntary saccades in relation to their amplitude. The amplitude of most such saccades lies between 1 and 25 minutes of angle. The minimal dimensions of these saccades are 2–5 minutes of angle. The maximal dimensions are approximately 40–50 minutes of angle. It should be noted that even minimal saccades of only 2–5 minutes of angle are strictly identical for both eyes (Fig. 64). Records show that the duration of the small involuntary saccades, depending on their amplitude, is 0.01–0.02 sec. This short duration (in conjunction with their small amplitude) is responsible for the fact that the saccades are completely

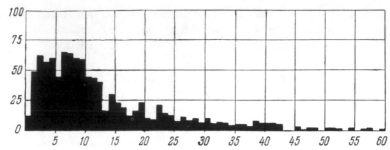

Fig. 63. Graph of distribution of 1000 involuntary horizontal saccades in accordance with their amplitude during fixation directed towards a stationary point. Results obtained with one subject.   Abscissa—amplitudes of saccades in minutes of angle; ordinate—number of approximately equal saccades.

unnoticed by the observer, to whom the fixation process appears to be continuous.

It has been found that an observer cannot voluntarily perform saccades smaller than a certain amplitude. In one experiment the subject was shown two fixation points separated by a distance of 8 minutes of angle. The problem was to fixate on the points alternately. The records showed that the saccades, and the alternation of the subject's attention from one point of fixation to the other (which appeared to the subject as alternation of the points of fixation) in most cases did not coincide in time. In other words, the subject could not change the point of fixation absolutely voluntarily when the distance between them was commensurate with the amplitude of the smallest involuntary

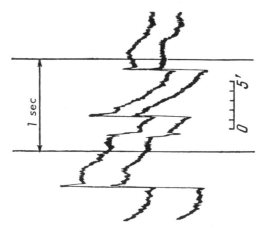

Fig. 64. Photokymographic record of eye movements during fixation on a stationary point. The record shows clearly that even the small saccades for the two eyes coincide in amplitude and direction.

saccades.   The subjective assessment of the moment of alternation of the points of fixation corresponded not to the times that saccades occurred, but to the times that attention was switched. In this case the subject controlled his attention but not his saccades.

Three cases may be noted when saccades are not associated with shift of attention. First, involuntary saccades arise when an observer tries to cast his eye smoothly around the outlines of a stationary object. Evidence of the existence of involuntary saccades in this case is given by records of the eye movements such as those shown in Fig. 53. Second, involuntary saccades arise during fixation on a stationary point when the duration of this fixation is longer than a certain time interval. A 5-minute record of fixation made on a stationary photographic film appears as an oval spot (which can be regarded as the projection of the foveola on the film). The study of records within this spot shows that many involuntary saccades occur when the image of the point of fixation lies in the center of the fovea, i.e., when there is no need for a correcting saccade (directing the image of the point of fixation to the center of the fovea). Finally, involuntary saccades arise when correction is necessary, i.e., when as a result of drift the image of the point of fixation begins to move outside or has moved outside the central region of the fovea. Such saccades are especially numerous in people

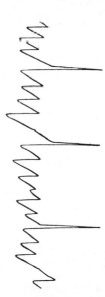

Fig. 65. Photokymographic record of the eye movement of a patient during fixation on a stationary point. In this case the drift of the patient's eye follows a direction, and the velocity of the drift is much higher than normal.

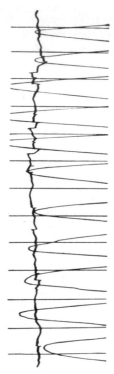

Fig. 66. Simultaneous recording on a photokymograph of the movements of the eye and rotations of the subject's head during fixation on a stationary point. During the experiment the subject continuously rotated his head from left to right and from right to left. The bold line is the record of the eye movements. The thin lines running on the edge of the figure are the records of the head movements.

with certain disturbances of the normal function of the muscular apparatus of the eye. By way of an example, a record made on a slit photokymograph by means of the P_1 cap with the patient trying to fixate on a stationary point is shown in Fig. 65. The drift of this patient's eye was directed to the right (the thick sloping lines), and the speed of the drift was higher than normal. Involuntary correcting saccades (thin horizontal lines) constantly returned the eye to its initial position.

4. FIXATION ON A POINT IN COMPLEX CONDITIONS

The simplest case—when the subject's head and the object of perception are stationary—was examined in the previous section. Conditions are much more complex for the observer's eye if fixation on a stationary object is accompanied by movement of the head, especially a rotary movement. In this case, the eyes must turn in the orbit smoothly so that, for a certain interval of time, the optical axes intersect the point of fixation. A fairly complex situation arises if the observer's head remains stationary, but the object of perception moves in space, so that the eyes must move continually to preserve fixation. Finally, another complex case is that which arises when both the observer's head and the visual test object move simultaneously.

Figures 66 and 67 will give some idea of the eye movements in complex conditions of fixation. Figure 66 shows a record of the eye movements during fixation while the subject was continuously rotating his head from left to right and from right to left. A record of the movement of both eyes when the subject fixated on a point performing oscillatory movements is shown in Fig. 67.

5. NYSTAGMUS OF THE EYES

In certain pathological cases, most frequently disorders of the nervous system, the process of fixation is accompanied by nystagmus. Nystagmus consists in an oscillatory movement of the axes of the eyes

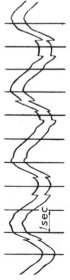

Fig. 67. Specimen of a photokymographic record of eye movements during pursuit of an object by means of oscillatory movements.

during which the amplitude of oscillation is tens of hundreds of times greater than the amplitude of the tremor, while the frequency of the nystagmus correspondingly is tens of times lower than the frequency of the tremor.

Different forms of nystagmus correspond to different forms of diseases. The same disease in different persons may be associated with the same or different types of nystagmus. As an example, several

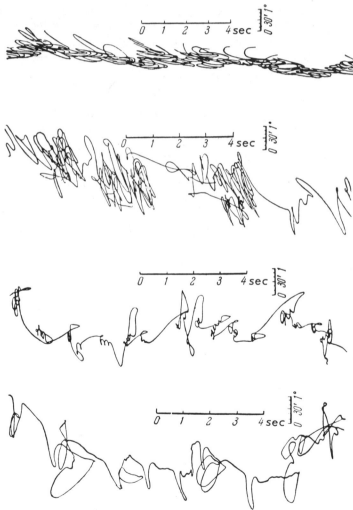

Fig. 68. Eye movements of rod monochromats T, A, O, and P during fixation on a point recorded on a vertically moving strip of photosensitive paper.

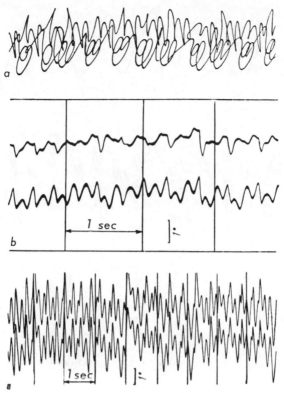

Fig. 69. Eye movements of rod monochromat T during fixation on a point. a) Horizontal movement of a strip of photosensitive paper; b) horizontal component of the movements recorded on a photokymograph; c) record of vertical component of the movements.

records of nystagmus in rod monochromat subjects are shown (the records were made on a photokymograph by means of the P_1 cap). In rod monochromats, only the rods are concerned in vision; the center of the fovea, occupied mainly by cones, does not function. The records in Fig. 68 show the eye movements of four rod monochromats as they attempt to fixate on a stationary point. These records show how different the types of nystagmus present in these four cases were. Nystagmus of the eyes of one rod monochromat is illustrated in Fig. 69. Finally, in Fig. 70, records of the eye movements of rod monochromats are given during fixation on an oscillating point.

Little study has yet been made of the various forms of nystagmus, although it is certainly possible that knowledge of the full range of varieties of this type of eye movement could be clinically useful. The vestibular forms of nystagmus arising in persons and in some animals

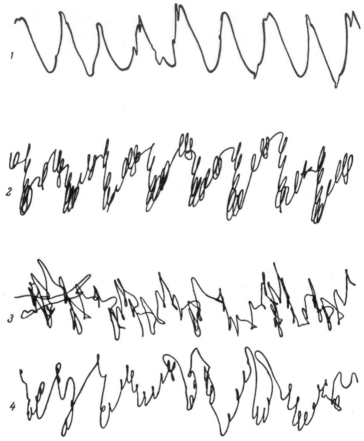

Fig. 70. Record of eye movements during pursuit of a moving sphere. 1) During pursuit of a sphere swinging on a thread by a subject with normal vision; 2) during pursuit by the rod monochromat person T of a sphere moving up and down; 3 and 4) during pursuit of a sphere swinging on a thread by the rod monochromat persons A and O. Movement of the tape is in a vertical direction.

in response to certain types of excitation of the vestibular apparatus have, however, been studied most intensively.

6. FACTORS INFLUENCING THE MOVEMENT AND CONTRAST OF THE RETINAL IMAGE

As mentioned earlier, movement of the retinal image over the retina and changes in this image itself during fixation are not determined only by the drift, tremor, and saccades of the eye. Many other factors besides these influence the movement and contrast of the retinal image.

The first point to mention is that in many cases the fixation process is interrupted by blinking movements of the eye, each lasting several tenths of a second. A blinking movement is accompanied by sharp changes in the illuminance of the retina and by disappearance of the retinal image for a certain period of time. While moistening the cornea with lachrymal fluid, the eyelid completely covers the pupil. In addition, during the blinking movement, the eyes make a small rotation and then return to their initial position (upward, medially, and back again), taking about 0.1-0.2 sec for one of these movements (Ginsborg, 1952).

Movements and rotations of the head, even if small and compensated to some extent by corresponding rotations of the eyes, always produce some displacement of the retinal image.

The position of the lens in the eye and the curvature of its surfaces do not remain strictly constant during fixation. The continuous movement of the lens is explained by the fact that it is a component of a self-adjusting system with continuous correction. The fluctuating changes

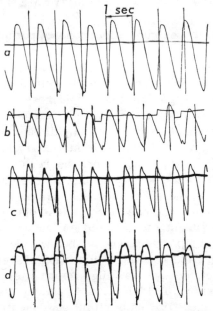

Fig. 71. Record of the pulsation of the eye. a) Healthy eye; b) eye of a patient with glaucoma (increased intraocular pressure; the higher the pressure, the smaller the amplitude); c and d) in patients with disturbances of the vascular system of the eye. The thick lines are records of eye movements, the thin lines record the pulsation.

thus produced in the parameters of the optical system of the eye lead to an irregular displacement of the retinal image and to a change in its sharpness. Although such changes are small, they nevertheless can be detected in some experiments with a stabilized image.

The constant, although small, change in the size of the pupil which takes place during fixation leads mainly to slight modulation of the brightness of the retinal image and to a change in the depth of focus. Many almost imperceptible and minor changes are brought about by the pulsation of the blood. For example, pulsating movements of the eye in the orbit (which differ in each individual) have been observed by means of relatively simple optical instruments and accessories. With the use of the P_5 cap, the pulsation of the eye itself has been recorded (Fig. 71). Measurements show that, as a result of pulsation, the curvature of the cornea changes by approximately one hundredth or several thousandths of a millimeter. Hence it is natural to suppose that the diameter of the eye as a whole may change considerably. Pulsating changes in the size of the eye evidently cause negligible changes in the sharpness of the fixed object.

7. ROLE OF EYE MOVEMENTS

As mentioned above, good conditions of perception require some degree of discrete or continuous movement of the retinal image over the retina, and the retinal image itself must possess adequate brightness and contrast. The experiments described in Chapter II showed that with a gradual slight increase or decrease in the luminance of a test field stationary relative to the retina the eye is able to distinguish between fairly small elements of the field, but cannot perceive color absolutely correctly. If a test field stationary relative to the retina is illuminated by a flickering light, the resolving power of the eye becomes so low that details with angular dimensions of a whole degree (and in some cases, of several degrees) can no longer be seen by the observer. All colors become more or less distorted in these conditions. In one experiment, the test field stationary relative to the retina was initially in complete darkness, but was later illuminated by a bright beam of light and remained illuminated thereafter. Although the resolving power of the eye was high immediately after the light was switched on, an empty field formed so quickly (sometimes within 1 second) that prolonged fixation of attention, essential in many cases of perception, was impossible.

Modulation of illumination in these conditions can delay the formation of an empty field or prevent its formation, but will always lead to distortion of visible colors and sometimes to a decrease in the resolving power of the eye. If a test field, stationary relative to the retina, is illuminated by a bright flash of light, the resolving power of the eye remains high but, just as in the preceding case, prolonged fixation of attention is impossible.

I conclude from these facts that good conditions for perception cannot be obtained if the retinal image is strictly stationary.

Let us try to examine in more detail the types of eye movement which are needed to create the essential conditions for perception during fixation of an element of a stationary object. The first fact to note is that ordinarily the end of a blinking movement or the end of any saccade (a large voluntary one or a small involuntary one) is always the beginning of a new process of seeing. I say "new" because I suggest that as a result of any blinking movement or saccade, certain signals arising from the retina are inhibited while others reappear. Ditchburn, Fender, and Mayne (1959) showed that even saccades of as little as 2.5 minutes of angle in magnitude reveal contours in a test field which have disappeared due to immobility of the retinal image (the minimal amplitude of the involuntary saccades arising during fixation is 2-5 minutes of angle).

It may be assumed that immediately after a blinking movement new signals arise from the whole retina, and immediately after a saccade (depending on the amplitude of the saccade and the type of object) new signals arise from the whole retina or from certain of its parts. Frequently situations arise when, after a saccade or series of saccades (especially if they are small), the changes in the illuminance of the receptors in certain parts of the retina are below the threshold required for signals to appear, in which case these areas will correspond to an empty field or to some stage in the formation of an empty field.

The spatial evolution of the fast process (the comet) shows that the initial stage of this process (immediately after a sharp change in illuminance) corresponds to optimal conditions of perception (the front, uniform part of the comet is always the brightest or blackest, the most saturated in color). It may therefore be considered that the maximal number of signals is sent to the visual centers immediately after a blinking movement or saccade.

Formation of an empty field, which may begin immediately after a blinking movement or saccade, would take place quickly and frequently much before the following saccade if the retinal image remained strictly stationary. This conclusion is based on the fact that the duration of the intensive part of the fast process does not exceed 1-3 seconds, while the duration of some drifts during fixation (Fig. 59) may amount to 5 or even 10 seconds. Experiments show that the drift of the eyes is the type of movement which prevents the formation of an empty field during fixation. Because of drift, the resolving power of the eye and the apparent color of the object show little change during fixation. In experiments to demonstrate the spatial evolution of the fast process, the following facts were established. If the image of the border between black and white fields moves over the retina at uniform velocity, and if this border is projected on the retina by means of an imperfect optical system, such as the optical system of the cap, in conditions of very bright illumination of the eye through the sclera, the border will be clearly visible to the subject if the velocity is not less than 23-24 minutes of angle per second. When such an experiment is carried out without illumination of the sclera, this border appears at velocities of 3-5 minutes of angle per second. On the other hand, records of eye drifts show that, although the mean velocity of this movement is 5-6 minutes of angle per second, frequently (not less than one or several times per second) it reaches almost maximal values, i.e., about 30 minutes of angle per second. Comparing these results it is easy to conclude that when sharp retinal images (sharp images of borders) are present, a single drift of the eye is sufficient to prevent the formation of an empty field over the whole retina.

An attempt was made to investigate the role of tremor using caps and several accessories. However, no effect of tremor on reception could be found. This is evidently due mainly to the fact that the principal frequency of tremor is much higher than the critical frequency of flicker fusion. If tremor has an effect on reception, it is only when combined with drift. The results of experiments in which I tried to discover as fully as possible the role of tremor unfortunately cannot be regarded as completely conclusive. For this reason, I shall not describe these experiments and shall leave the question of tremor open.

Ditchburn, Fender, and Mayne (1959) found that low-frequency tremor has a positive influence on discrimination of the elements of a test field stationary relative to the retina. In this investigation tremor was produced artificially with frequencies ranging from 4 to 20 oscillations per second and with an amplitude of between 0.05 and 1.10 minutes of angle. They found that for all the investigated frequencies of tremor with an amplitude exceeding 0.3 minute of angle, the fraction of time for which the subject saw the test object was increased. However, the artificial tremor created by these authors has little in common with natural tremor in its frequency or character of movement, for logically, tremor is best defined as only the high-frequency (over 40 cps) component of the movement of the eye relative to the orbit. Natural tremor is characterized by a frequency higher than the critical frequency of flicker fusion. Low frequencies during fixation should be classified as drifts.

During fixation, besides the drifts of the eye, any other factor causing movement of the retinal image over the retina may prevent formation of an empty field. For example, if a sharp retinal image is shifted for several tenths of a second through several minutes of angle because of head movements, no empty field will form. In natural conditions of perception, the fixation process is constantly accompanied by movements of several types. As records show, it is difficult to accept that the sum of these movements does not exceed the frequency required for good conditions of perception even by as little as one per second. Hence, under natural conditions, it is almost impossible to make an empty field appear even when the observer wishes. Such an attempt is usually successful only for very short periods of time and only if the retinal image is highly out of focus.

CONCLUSIONS

Fixation of attention directed towards an element of a stationary object is accompanied by fixation of the gaze. Subjectively, this fixation of the gaze is perceived by the observer as fixation by stationary eyes.

In reality, however, the eye moves in three ways during fixation: by small involuntary saccades, equal for the two eyes; by drift, slow, irregular movement of the optical axes in which, however, some degree of constancy of their position is retained; and by tremor, an oscillatory movement of the axes of the eyes of high frequency but low amplitude.

Head movements, blinking movements of the eyes, saccades, drift, and tremor during fixation on an element of a stationary object create a certain mobility of the retinal image and prevent the formation of an empty field.

The formation of an empty field in intervals between saccades is prevented mainly by the drift of the eyes.

Chapter IV

SACCADIC EYE MOVEMENTS

As mentioned above, two features are characteristic of any saccadic movement of the eyes: (1) an almost perfect identity of the
movements of both eyes; and (2) high velocity (the duration of saccades
is measured in hundredths of a second). Under normal conditions these
features are constantly observed and may be clearly recorded by any
suitably sensitive method of studying eye movements.

The main function of saccades is to change the points of fixation, to
direct the most sensitive region of the retina (the fovea) to a particular
element of the object of perception. The nature of saccades is responsible for much of the refinement of perception. The high velocity
and correspondingly short duration of the saccades usually permit the
eye to remain in a state of fixation for about 95% of the total time.

The velocity and duration of the saccades were first studied by
Lamansky (1869) who used the method of after-images. During the
experiment, when the points of fixation were changed, a bright flickering source of light was kept in the subject's field of vision. Every
time the change of points of fixation was complete, the light was turned
off, and the subject perceived the after-image in the form of a broken
line. Given the flicker frequency and the number of flashes imprinted
during the change in the points of fixation, the experimenter could
determine approximately the duration and velocity of the saccade.
Saccades have also been studied in detail by Dodge (1907) and more
recently by A. L. Yarbus (1956c), Westheimer (1958), and B. Kh.
Gurevich (1961).

1. DURATION OF THE SACCADE

Let us first consider in detail the question of the duration of the
saccades. In all experiments to record saccades, the P_1 cap was used

together with a special slit photokymograph, in which the photosensitive paper moved at a speed of 5 m/sec. The photosensitive paper was fixed to the large and rapidly turning drum of the photokymograph. During the experiments the subject was shown two points equidistant from the axis of the cyclopic eye; he fixated alternately on the two points. The distance between the points of fixation varied from experiment to experiment. The amplitude of the saccades was determined entirely from the records on the photokymograph paper, since the angular measurement of the saccades differed systematically from the angular distance between the points intended for fixation (usually the angular measurement of the saccade was less than the angular distance between these points). Because of the high velocity of movement of the photosensitive paper, the duration of the saccades could be measured with an accuracy of ±0.01 sec.

Some idea of the character of the eye movements during a saccade may be gained from the records shown in Fig. 72 of horizontal saccades between two points visible to the observer at an angle of 8°. It is clear from Fig. 72 that during a change in the points of fixation the velocity of the eye movement rises smoothly, reaches a maximum, and then falls smoothly.

In natural conditions the amplitude of the saccade usually does not exceed 20°. Very often rotations of the eyes exceeding 15° may be composed of two or three saccades, or they may even be accompanied by a corresponding rotation of the head. Lancaster (1941) claims that about 99% of eye movements are composed of saccades less than 15° in amplitude.

Later we shall study saccades whose amplitude does not exceed 20°. In the first series of experiments the duration of horizontal saccades was measured. The results of these experiments are given in Fig. 73. The duration of vertical saccadic eye movements is illustrated in Fig. 74. The same results are shown in Fig. 75 for saccades taking place at an angle of 45° to the horizontal (or vertical) plane.

The following conclusions may be drawn from an examination of Figs. 73, 74, and 75. The duration of the saccade is dependent on its amplitude; for saccades measuring only a few degrees, the duration lies between 0.01 and 0.02 sec, while for saccades of 20° it may exceed 0.07 sec. The duration of the saccade is independent of or only slightly dependent on, the direction in which it occurs. This conclusion is drawn from the fact that the graphs in Figs. 73, 74, and 75 differ only slightly from each other. It is clear from the graphs (Figs. 73, 74, and 75) that saccades of the same size may vary in duration. The durations of the saccades of the same amplitude may differ by as much

as 0.01, or even 0.015 second in duration. The next experiments
examined the question of whether the duration of the saccade depends
on the position of the eye at the moment the saccade begins   It was
found that, apart from the most extreme positions (positions of the eye
not found in natural conditions of perception), the duration of the saccade depends entirely on its amplitude and is not appreciably dependent
on the position from which this saccade is performed. To confirm this
conclusion, the results of one series of experiments are given in
Fig. 76.   The graph in this figure shows the durations of the vertical
and horizontal saccades made by a subject in a number of unusual
conditions.   Vertical saccades were performed when the eye was
turned downward almost to the limit, and horizontal saccades were
performed when the eye was turned to the left almost to the limit. The
distance between the points of fixation in both cases was 3°. It is easy
to see that the duration of the saccades and their scatter in this case
do not differ substantially from the duration and scatter of the saccades
of the same amplitude illustrated in Figs. 73, 74, and 75.

Attempts were next made to determine the extent to which the duration of the saccade depends on the subject's will, and whether, for
example, a subject can perform saccades of the same angular magnitude

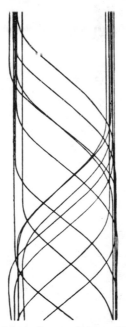

Fig. 72. Sample recording of saccades on photosensitive paper moving at 5m/sec.

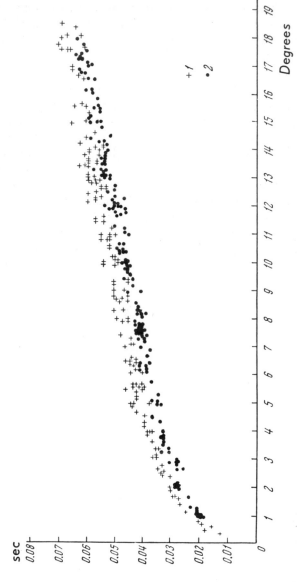

Fig. 73. Graph of duration (in seconds) of horizontal saccades of the eye as a function of the angle (in degrees) through which the eye turned when changing the points of fixation. 1) Subject K; 2) subject P.

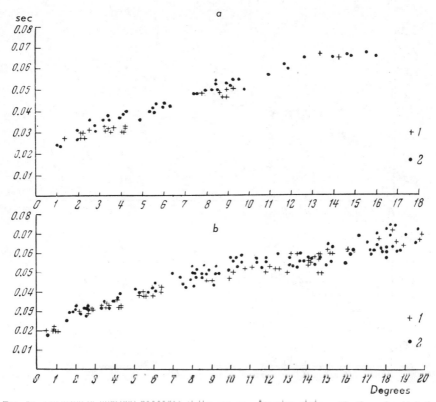

Fig. 74. Duration of vertical saccades of the eye as a function of the angle through which the eye turned when changing the points of fixation. a) Subject P; b) subject R: 1) Readings obtained while subject's eye was moving upward; 2) the same, while the eye was moving downward.

at different speeds, thus changing their duration. The records showed that a subject cannot voluntarily change the duration and character of the saccade. Usually, all the subjects felt that it was relatively easy to make the saccades faster or slower at will. However, the records showed that the sensation of a fast saccade appears as a result of a decreased duration of fixation on the points between which the saccade is made. All attempts to make fast saccades were accompanied by a reduced (compared with the normal) duration of fixation. Attempts to make slow saccades produced a very brief intermediate stop (0.1-0.2 sec). In other words, a subject trying to make a particular saccade slow, made instead two or three ordinary saccades of smaller amplitude. The intermediate stop in this case was not noticed by the subject, so that the changes in the points of fixation appeared to be slow. The duration of saccades, some of which subjects tried to make

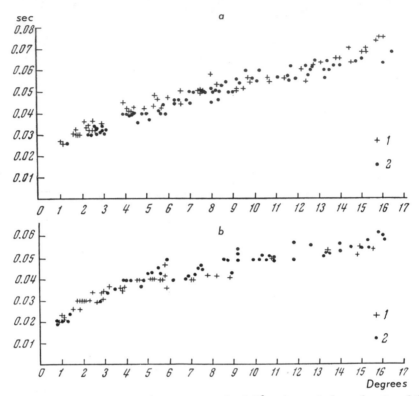

Fig. 75. Duration of saccades of the eye at an angle of 45° to the vertical as a function of the angle through which the eye turned when changing the points of fixation. a) Subject K; b) subject R: 1) Readings obtained when the subject's eyes moved upward and to the right; 2) when the eyes moved downward and to the left.

very fast and others very slow, is illustrated in Fig. 77. It is clear from this figure that for each of the three subjects some of the "fast" saccades lasted longer than the "slow." From experiments such as these it is concluded that, generally speaking, after the parameters of a saccade have been assigned and the saccade has begun, it cannot be modified in any way.

Besides the experiments described above, other considerations favor this view. Since saccades last only several hundredths of a second, it is hard to believe that any form of correction can be introduced into their course, or that the amplitude of the saccade can be changed during such short intervals of time. Experiments show that any corrections to saccades, when they occur (as they very often do), take place by means of small supplementary saccades, but only after the primary saccade is completed. At the time of a saccade, the

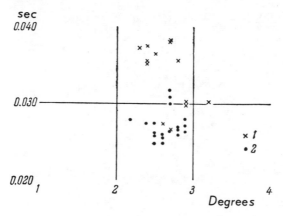

Fig. 76. Duration of saccades. Fixation points given at an angle of 3°. 1) Readings made while the eyes were turned downward almost to the limit. Vertical saccades; 2) readings made while the eyes were turned to the left almost to the limit. Horizontal saccades.

angular velocity of movement of the eyes is so great that in perception of stationary objects the retinal image may be regarded as "blurred." Because of this blurring we usually see nothing during a saccade, and it is highly improbable that in such conditions the eye should be able to receive information necessary for introducing any form of correction.

The duration of saccades made by the eyes of several observers is shown in Fig. 78. From such graphs an attempt was made to discover individual variations in the saccades of different observers. It may be concluded from an examination of the graph in Fig. 73 and graph *a*

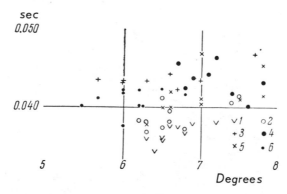

Fig. 77. Duration of saccades of the eye when the observer tried to make fast or slow saccades. Fixation points given at an angle of 7°. Subject K: 1) "fast" saccades; 2) "slow". Subject P: 3) "fast" saccades; 4) "slow." Subject R: 5) "fast" saccades; 6) "slow."

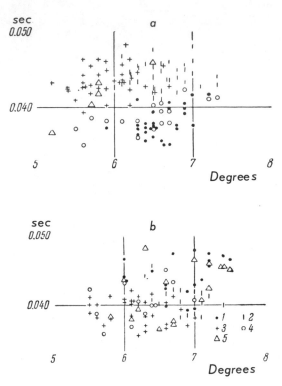

Fig. 78. Duration of saccades of five subjects. Fixation points given at an angle of 7°. a—Graph of duration of horizontal saccades; b—duration of vertical saccades. 1) Subject K; 2) subject P; 3) subject R; 4) subject KN; 5) subject T.

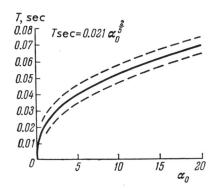

Fig. 79. Graph showing relationship between duration of the saccade and the angle through which the eye turns.

in Fig. 78 that the duration of the horizontal saccades differs slightly from one observer to another (by several thousandths of a second). However, graph *b* in Fig. 78, showing the duration of the vertical saccades, does not have this clear difference. Hence individual variations in the duration of saccades in different subjects must not be taken for granted; in many cases this variation may evidently be disregarded.

It is clear from Figs. 76, 77, and 78 that, on the average, the amplitude of the saccades is less than the angular distance between the points of fixation. For example, when the distance between the points of fixation was 7° (Figs. 77 and 78), the mean amplitude of the saccades performed between these points was 6.5°. The experiments show that this phenomenon is always encountered if the object of fixation consists of points. If two clearly visible and large enough vertical lines are drawn through two such points, for example on the horizontal plane, the records show that the amplitudes of the saccades will not coincide with the angular distance between the vertical lines in this case either.

Summarizing the data in section 1, it may be said that under normal conditions the duration of the saccadic movements of the eyes is, roughly speaking, only a function of the angle through which the eye turns when changing the points of fixation. The relationship between the duration of the saccade and the angle through which the eye turns may be expressed by the following empirical formula (Fig. 79):

$$T = 0.021 \, a_0^{2/5}$$

where T is the duration of the saccade in seconds, and a_0 the angle in degrees through which the eye turns when changing the points of fixation. The maximal scatter of the experimental points (Fig. 79) is approximately ±0.005–0.007 sec.

2. DEVELOPMENT OF THE SACCADE IN TIME

Careful examination of the records of saccades in Fig. 72 will reveal the close resemblance between these records and sinusoidal curves. Closer examination shows that in fact the records of most horizontal and vertical saccades not exceeding 15–20° approximate sinusoids very nearly (oblique saccades are not now being considered). As an example, records of horizontal saccades with the points of the corresponding sinusoid marked directly on the paper tape of the photokymograph are shown in Fig. 80. Records of saccades measuring

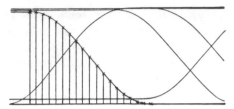

Fig. 80. Records of saccades. The points of the corresponding sinusoid are plotted on one of the tracings.

15-20° show a much less close approximation to the sinusoidal curve. In the middle part of the curve, rectilinear areas appear (corresponding to uniform velocity), and the curves become slightly asymmetrical (the time of increase in velocity of the saccade is apparently shorter than the time of its decrease). According to some authors (Hyde, 1959), this asymmetry is particularly noticeable with very large saccades (50-60°). Naturally, therefore, recordings of saccades larger than 15-20° cannot approximate a sinusoid. For saccades of less than 15-20°, we can give a formula describing the change in the angle of rotations of the eye during the saccade in time (Fig. 81):

$$\alpha = \frac{a_0}{2}\left(1-\cos\frac{\pi}{T}\,t\right), \tag{1}$$

where t is the time in seconds, $(0 < t < T)$, α is the angle of rotation during the saccade in degrees $(0 << \alpha << a_0)$, T is the duration of the saccade in seconds, and a_0 is the amplitude of the saccade in degrees.

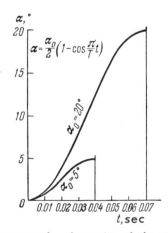

Fig. 81. Relationship between angle of rotation of the eye and time during a saccade.

By differentiating equation (1), we obtain a formula for the angular velocity (ω) of the eye movement during a saccade (Fig. 82):

$$\omega = \frac{da}{dt} = \frac{a_0 t}{2T} \sin \frac{\pi}{T} t. \tag{2}$$

Naturally this formula only approximately describes the course of saccades measuring 15–20° and it cannot be applied to saccades larger than 20°.

Assuming that the radius of the eye is 1.2 cm, and using formula (2), we obtain an expression for the linear velocities (v) of the center of the cornea in the process of a saccade not exceeding 20° in amplitude (Fig. 82).

$$v = 0.021 \, \omega. \tag{3}$$

It follows from equation (2) that the velocity of the saccade rises smoothly, reaches a maximum, and then falls smoothly to zero. For saccades smaller than 15–20°, the increase and decrease of velocity follow a sinusoidal rule (the times of increase and decrease in velocity are approximately equal). For large saccades (exceeding 20°) the increase in velocity occupies less than half the total duration of the saccade. A correspondingly longer period of time is occupied by the decrease in the velocity of the saccade. The maximal velocities of the saccades are clearly dependent on their amplitude.

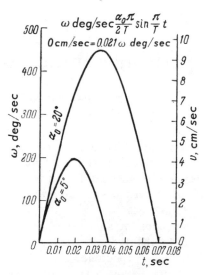

Fig. 82. Relationship between angular and linear velocity of eye movement and time during a saccade.

For example, for a saccade of 5°, the eye reaches a maximal velocity of 200 deg/sec, and for a saccade of 20°, about 450 deg/sec. The study of records similar to those shown in Fig. 72 demonstrates that maximal acceleration during saccadic movements is attained by the eye at the very beginning of the saccade and at its end (at the end, the acceleration has the opposite sign, slowing the saccade).

The absolute magnitudes of the two accelerations for small saccades are almost identical, but for large saccades (exceeding 20°), they differ considerably (the acceleration at the beginning of the saccade is greater than the acceleration at its end).

The magnitude of the accelerations clearly depends on the amplitude of the saccade. For example, for a saccade of 5° it is approximately 15,000 deg/sec^2, and for a saccade of 20° about 20,000 deg/sec^2.

Disregarding friction between the eye and the orbit, regarding the eye as a sphere and the vitreous and the other intraocular media as rigidly fixed to the sclera, and knowing the accelerations, it is easy to calculate the forces setting the eye in motion during the saccade. Assuming that the radius of the eye is 1.2 cm and its specific gravity is 1, we obtain that the maximal effort of the muscles at the beginning of a saccade of 5° is approximately 1 g, and that at the beginning of a saccade of 20° about 1.5 g. When considering this ideal case, we must naturally remember that the eye does not turn in a medium of air but in the orbit. For this reason, even assuming that muscular effort is used up only in rotating the eye, in this case it must be considerably larger than the forces indicated in these examples.

3. INCLINATION OF SACCADES

Many experiments have shown that saccades in a horizontal or vertical direction are in most cases recorded on stationary photosensitive paper as straight lines. Saccades performed at an angle to these two directions are most frequently recorded as curved lines. Two questions arise in this connection: what is the reason for this curvature of the lines; and to what extent can we apply our conclusions regarding horizontal and vertical saccades to oblique saccades   Let us first turn to Figs. 83 and 84.

Figure 83 shows records of saccades between all corners of two equal squares situated in the frontal plane. The records were made with the P_1 cap on stationary photosensitive paper. One square was placed so that two of its sides were horizontal and the other two vertical. The other square was so placed that all its sides made an

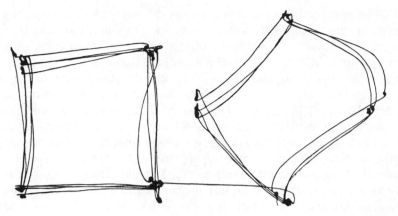

Fig. 83. Record of saccades between the corners of two squares on stationary photosensitive paper.

angle of 45° with the horizontal. The sharp differences between the records of the saccades in these two cases are clear from Fig. 83.

To determine whether the curvature of the oblique saccades is due to rotary (around the geometrical axis) movements of the eyes, an experiment was carried out using the P_1 cap with the mirror in an unusual position. The mirror was fixed to the cap so that it was in the sagittal plane during the experiment. In other words, it was parallel to the vertical section passing through the axis of the eye, and its reflecting surface was directed towards the temple. The source of light and the photosensitive material (the photographic paper) were arranged correspondingly on the temporal side.

During the experiment the subject was asked to make several saccades with his eyes between all the corners of the two squares situated in the frontal plane, as described in the previous experiment. This time the position of the mirror was so arranged that only the horizontal movement of the eye and rotary movements of the eyes around the geometrical axis (or, roughly speaking, around the optic axis) could be recorded on the photosensitive paper. The vertical movements could not be reproduced. The results of this experiment are shown in Fig. 84.

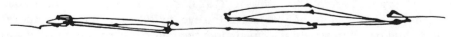

Fig. 84. Saccades between the corners of two squares on stationary photosensitive paper recorded when only the horizontal components of the movements and the rotary movements of the eye around the optic axis could be recorded.

When performing saccades between the corners of the squares, the eye performed eight different movements: two in a vertical direction (up and down), two in a horizontal direction (from left to right and from right to left), and four in various oblique directions. These results suggest that under normal conditions, when the observer's head and the object of perception are stationary, no appreciable movements are observed around the geometrical axis of the eye, and, consequently, the curvature of the lines obtained by recording oblique saccades cannot be attributed to rotary (around the geometrical axis) movements of the eyes. The curvature of oblique saccades may take place as a result of the nonsimultaneous working of the different muscles. We may note, incidentally, that fairly considerable rotary movements of the eyes (around the orbit) may be observed in conditions when the subject examines a stationary object, and when so doing turns his head around the axis of the cyclopic eye.

If two harmonic oscillations are superposed at an angle, curvilinear trajectories known as Lissajous figures are obtained. Since the records of horizontal and vertical saccades (less than 15-20°) approximate a sinusoid, the possibility remains that the records of oblique saccades consist mainly of Lissajous figures.

Naturally, when applied to oblique saccades, the equations given in the preceding section are observed less accurately than for horizontal and vertical saccades. However, as Fig. 75 shows, the duration of oblique saccades is indistinguishable from the duration of horizontal and vertical saccades of the same amplitude. Analysis of the records of oblique saccades (analysis of the component along the straight line connecting the points of fixation) also shows that along the straight line connecting the points of fixation all the characteristics of oblique saccades are almost indistinguishable from the corresponding characteristics of horizontal or vertical saccades. For this reason, in calculations of practical importance, any saccades (not exceeding 15-20°) of the same amplitude can usually be regarded as equal in all respects.

4. CENTER OF ROTATION OF THE EYE

George, Toren, and Löwell (1923) demonstrated that in a zone bounded by the angle of rotation of the eye by 20° towards the temporal side and by 30° towards the nasal side, the center of rotation of the eye may be regarded as a fixed point situated 15.4 mm from the apex of the cornea and 1.65 mm to the nasal side of the optic axis. Outside

Table 1

Direction of optic axis	39° towards nose	4° towards nose	38° towards temple
Distance of center of rotation from apex of cornea, mm	14.73	13.92	12.95
Distance of center of rotation from optic axis, mm	1.066	1.653	0.893

the limits of this zone the center of rotation of the eye, according to these workers, is no longer fixed. Park and Park (1933) repeated these observations and obtained the results as to the localization of the center of rotation of the eye for three directions, as shown in Table 1.

These results (even if of doubtful accuracy) show that, for the majority of eye movements (excluding rotations through angles greater than 20-30°), the center of rotation of the eye may be regarded as a stationary point. However, the possibility remains (Lord and Wright, 1950) that this center may be displaced and may even lie outside the eye itself during certain small saccades. Such a displacement may arise, for example, if a saccade is accompanied by linear displacement of the eye relative to the orbit.

5. BEGINNING AND END OF THE SACCADE

Normally, for the perception of stationary objects the eye must be in one of two states—in a state of fixation or in the process of changing the points of fixation. Let us examine the eye movements during the transition from fixation to the process of changing the points of fixation, and vice versa. So as not to anticipate the issue, let us exclude from our examination the case where points of fixation are shifted during pursuit or at moments of convergence or divergence of the eyes. The many records which have been made show that the transition from a state of fixation to a saccade (for horizontal and vertical saccades of less than 15-20°) may be expressed by equation (1) in section 2. As a rule this equation is valid not only for the main part of the saccade, but also for its beginning, lasting for the first few milliseconds. The transition from the state of the saccade to the state of fixation (lasting for the last few milliseconds) cannot always be expressed by equation (1) in section 2, even for small saccades. Some delay in slowing of

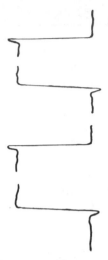

Fig. 85. Record of a change in the points of fixation on a slit photokymograph. The overshoot of the eye is clearly visible on the records.

the saccade is frequently observed, as a result of which the eye apparently shoots past the point at which it will stop at the next moment, but then returns to it (without a correcting saccade). A series of these overruns is shown in Fig. 85. It should be noted that different subjects overshoot by different amounts. In the same subject, some saccades terminate by overshooting, while others show this tendency hardly at all. The degree of overshoot is independent, or almost independent, of the amplitude of the saccade. In normal con- ditions, by comparison with the large saccades, the overshoot is so slight that it can almost be disregarded. Often, by comparison with small involuntary saccades, the overshoot is considerable; it is espe- cially significant for saccades resembling tremor of the eyes (tremor of the eyes during fixation).

6. VISION DURING THE SACCADE

During perception of stationary objects, at the moment of the saccade no visual images are formed because the high velocity of the retinal image leads to "blurring" of everything falling within the field of vision. We can observe this "blurring," for example, if we look at the road with a fixed glance from the window of a fast moving automobile, or if we examine a rotating disk.

The question may arise: is this the only cause preventing the appearance of a visual image during a saccade? Is there no special type of inhibition arising concurrently with the saccade and excluding vision during its course? Several very simple experiments give a negative answer to this question. One such experiment is as follows. A large disk is placed before the observer. Along the perimeter of the disk is drawn or glued a large, periodically repeated pattern. For example, pieces of white paper may be glued along the perimeter of a dark disk. The disk is then turned at a speed at which, while the observer fixes his gaze on the edge of the disc, the patterns completely merge. If the observer then changes his points of fixation in the direction of movement of the patterns so that the angular velocities of the movements of the eyes and of the pattern are very close, for very short intervals of time (during the saccade) he will clearly see the patterns on the disk. Consequently, it can be concluded that during the saccade the eye does not lose its perceptive power; if the eye sees nothing, it is simply because it has to deal with a retinal image moving at high speed.

Examination of the evolution of the after-image in a completely darkened room reveals the following curious fact: nearly every saccadic movement of the eyes, if large enough, is accompanied by the temporary disappearance of the after-image, if it is weak; or by a change in its color if it is strong. The important thing here is that the temporary disappearance of the after-image lasts much longer than the saccade. Is this disappearance of the after-image due to some weak, partial inhibition of perception coinciding with the time of the saccades? (I say partial inhibition because, as we have seen, complete inhibition evidently does not occur.) The apparent color of the after-image may change suddenly in response to a change in the illuminance of the eye. In a totally dark room, however, the illuminance is zero.

In this case, therefore, only conjecture is possible; it could be that during the time of the saccade the effect I have mentioned is caused by a very slight dynamic shift of the intraocular media relative to the sclera. The shift may be too small to evoke movement phosphene, but sufficient to influence the apparent color of the after-image.

7. VOLUNTARY AND INVOLUNTARY SACCADES

In the preceding chapter we discussed the small involuntary saccades accompanying fixation on a stationary object. Such small saccades are unnoticed and cannot be produced at will.

It was mentioned above that even large saccades, those by means of which we change our direction of fixation, may be either involuntary or voluntary. There is much factual evidence to show that many large saccades are involuntary. For example, immediately after having examined an object we can say only approximately on which of its elements we fixed. The observer is in an extremely difficult position if he is asked to estimate, even approximately, the number of saccades performed in a very short period of time. He can easily perform large, voluntary saccades if he is asked to do so, for example, in the conditions of a particular experiment. In natural conditions of perception, even a shift of attention is not always voluntary, and the saccades accompanying the perception process are mainly unnoticed by the observer. Usually changes of attention remain in our memory, but not changes of points of fixation.

When we have learned to walk we do not think which foot to move first, we simply walk. When we have learned to look we do not think about what order or what points of fixation to choose when looking at an object, we simply look. But both in walking and in looking at objects, the "simplicity" of the movements is really very complex. The change of the points of fixation and the choice of these points take place in accordance with certain general principles which will be examined fully below. Here I shall merely mention that even saccades which are certainly voluntary are not always or entirely submissive to our will.

CONCLUSIONS

Any saccade of the eyes (a sharp rotation of the optic axes) shows characteristically an almost ideal identity of the movements of both eyes, and a high velocity. The main purpose of the saccades is to change the points of fixation, to change the direction of the most highly developed region of the retina (the fovea) to a particular element of the object of perception. Under natural conditions of perception, the amplitude of the saccades usually does not exceed 20°. Saccades of minimal amplitude measure 2-5 minutes of angle. The duration of the saccade changes with a change in its amplitude. For angles less than 1° the duration of the saccades is 0.01-0.02 sec; for angles of 20° it may reach 0.06-0.07 sec. The maximal velocity reached by the eye during a saccade of 20° is about 450 deg/sec. Under normal conditions, the duration of equal saccades in different observers is approximately the same; it cannot be varied at will by the observer and is determined almost entirely by the amplitude of the saccade.

Chapter V

EYE MOVEMENTS DURING CHANGE OF STATIONARY POINTS OF FIXATION IN SPACE

If points of fixation are removed to various distances from an observer's eyes, the change is accompanied not only by a saccade, but by convergence of the eyes (convergence or divergence of the optical axes). Together with accommodation (and other factors), the relative position of the optical axes and the retinal images enables us at moments of fixation to judge the distance and size of objects. In this book there is no need to dwell in detail on questions of binocular vision; the necessary information can be obtained from other sources—the book by S. V. Kravkov (1950), for example. The important issue so far as we are concerned is that the convergence and divergence of the optical axes during a change in points of fixation differ sharply from saccades, particularly in duration. The duration of convergence and divergence of the eyes is approximately ten times that of saccades. Convergence or divergence of the eyes very often is equal in duration to fixation.

It may be assumed that the considerable difference between the duration of saccades and that of convergence or divergence is due to the fact that the saccade follows a predetermined program, whereas the program for convergence and divergence cannot be laid down beforehand.

1. CHANGE OF STATIONARY POINTS OF FIXATION IN SPACE

Let us first attempt to explain the general character of eye movements during change of stationary points of fixation in space. I have

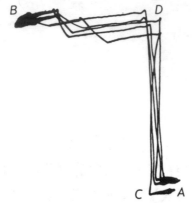

Fig. 86. Record of divergence of the left eye of a subject on stationary photosensitive paper during a change of stationary points of fixation. Both points of fixation are situated in the sagittal plane. The more distant point (B) is higher than the nearer point (A).

already remarked that this change is composed of two types of movements—the convergence or divergence of the optical axes and the saccade. More specifically, it is possible to change the points of fixation in space in such a way that there is no need to rotate the eye; the change then will consist purely of convergence or divergence. In the subsequent pages we shall study the general case of this type of movement.

Let us examine Figs. 86-88. From the records of eye movements shown in these figures, it is clear that a change in points of fixation in space is composed of two types of movement, and that a saccade of the eyes is always preceded by an initial stage of convergence or diver-

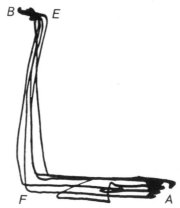

Fig. 87. Record of convergence of the left eye of a subject on stationary photosensitive paper during a change of stationary points of fixation. Both points of fixation are situated in the sagittal plane. The more distant point (B) is higher than the nearer point (A).

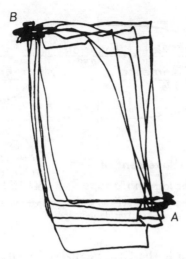

Fig. 88. Record of the movements of a subject's left eye during alternation of two points of fixation situated in the sagittal plane. The more distant point (B) is higher than the nearer point (A).

gence.   In the analogous experiments illustrated in Figs. 86, 87, and 88, the points of fixation (A and B) were white balls arranged in the sagittal plane relative to the subject in such a way that point B was further away and slightly above point A. The angular dimensions of the balls were 2°.   The P_1 cap was used in all experiments.   The minimal distance between the subject's eyes and point A was 15 cm, and the maximal distance to point B 950 cm.   The eye movements were recorded on stationary photosensitive paper in front of the subject. One of the records from the subject's left eye during five successive changes from point of fixation A to point of fixation B is shown in Fig. 86; the record from the right eye (relative to the sagittal plane) in this case was a mirror image of the record from the left eye.

All the records, which were similar to that shown in Fig. 86, showed that a change of the points of fixation (from point A to point B) follow the same scheme.   In the first period there is very slight divergence (AC), after which the eye performs a saccade in the direction of point B (CD), and after the saccade the main part of the divergence (DB) takes place.   If the fixation points are far apart and the saccade of the eyes is not accurate enough, often the second phase of divergence (DB) is accompanied by additional correcting saccades of the eyes.   Such corrective saccades can be seen in Fig. 86.

A record of the movements of the left eye during a change from point of fixation B to point of fixation A is shown in Fig. 87. Slight con-

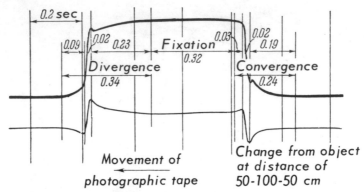

Fig. 89. Record of movements of both eyes on a photokymograph during a change of points of fixation in space.

vergence is observed in the first period (BE), after which the eye per-forms a saccade in the direction of point A (EF); and after the saccade, the main part of the convergence (FA) takes place and is sometimes accompanied by additional corrective saccades.   In Fig. 88 are shown the movements of a subject's left eye during successive changes in points of fixation from A to B and B to A.   In Fig. 89 is shown a record, made by means of a slit photokymograph, of the movements of both eyes during a change in points of fixation.   It is clear from this figure that

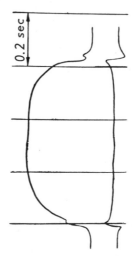

Fig. 90. Record of movements of both eyes on a photokymograph during a change of points of fixation in space. A case of asymmetrical eye movements during convergence and diver-gence.

convergence and divergence begin and end smoothly. In most cases the eye movements are different during convergence and divergence (Figs. 89 and 90).

The convergence and divergence of the optical axes may continue for several tenths of a second. The eyes perform smooth and slow convergence or divergence during the initial and final segments of this time (Figs. 89 and 90). The experiments show that a normal process of perception is possible during these segments of time (there is no duplication of the visual objects). In general, some degree of convergence and divergence of the optical axes during fixation does not cause duplication of visible objects (Kravkov, 1950); because of this, part of the time occupied by convergence and divergence of the eyes can at the same time be employed for perception. This fraction of the time is particularly large when the convergence or divergence of the optical axes is very slight.

Frequently the maximal angular velocity of the eye movement during convergence or divergence may attain several tens of degrees per second. Naturally, with these speeds, normal perception is no longer possible.

Simple experiments show that the eyes remain capable of perception at the moment of convergence or divergence (as during a saccade).

2. DURATION OF CONVERGENCE AND DIVERGENCE

In a large series of experiments using several subjects, the duration of convergence and divergence was measured. The P_1 cap was used in these experiments. Records were made simultaneously from both eyes on a slit photokymograph. The results of the measurements are shown in Fig. 91. The dots inside each column denote the duration of convergence, corresponding to a change in points of fixation situated at the following distances (in cm) from the subject's eyes: $25 \rightarrow 15$, $35 \rightarrow 25$, $45 \rightarrow 35$, and so on.

The x's inside each column denote the duration of divergence, corresponding to a change in points of fixation situated at the following distances (in cm) from the subject's eyes: $15 \rightarrow 25$, $25 \rightarrow 35$, $35 \rightarrow 45$, etc.

The results of the experiments illustrated in Fig. 91 demonstrate that the duration of convergence and divergence is measured in tenths of a second. By way of comparison it is well to recall that the duration of the saccades is measured in hundredths of a second. Under identical conditions, the duration of convergence may differ considerably (sometimes one may be twice the other). On the average, the duration of

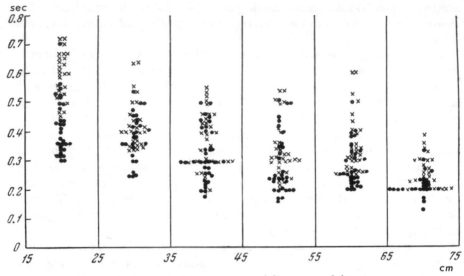

Fig. 91. Duration of convergence and divergence of the eyes.

divergence is slightly longer than the duration of convergence.

The duration of convergence and divergence of healthy eyes of different subjects is approximately equal and is not appreciably dependent on the subject's will to make these movements faster or slower.

In one series of experiments, conditions were created in which a new object of fixation appeared unexpectedly before the subject. The subject's task was to begin fixating on the new object immediately. Measurements showed that under these conditions the character and duration of covergence and divergence were indistinguishable from those observed in the previous experiments.

3. CONVERGENCE AND DIVERGENCE PRECEDING A SACCADE

As demonstrated above, during a change of stationary points of fixation in space, the saccade is always preceded by an initial stage of convergence or divergence. In a series of experiments similar to that described above, the duration of these initial stages was measured; these measurements are shown in Fig. 92. The dots inside each column denote the duration of the initial stages of convergence during a change in points of fixation situated at the following distances (in cm) from the subject's eyes: $25 \rightarrow 15$, $35 \rightarrow 25$, $45 \rightarrow 35$, and so on. The x's inside each column denote the duration of the initial stages of divergence during change in points of fixation situated at the following distances from the subject's eyes: $15 \rightarrow 25$, $25 \rightarrow 35$, $35 \rightarrow 45$ cm, and so on. Naturally, in these experiments two adjacent points of fixation were always slightly displaced relative to the axis of the subject's cyclopic eye, so that a change from one to the other would be accompanied by a saccade.

It is clear from the data in Fig. 92 that with any change of stationary points of fixation in space the duration of the process of convergence or divergence preceding the saccade is between 0.07 and 0.2 sec, and that this value is roughly constant. Since the preparation for a saccade to an object suddenly appearing in the subject's field of vision or preparation for pursuit of a suddenly appearing object takes 0.15-0.17 sec, it can be concluded that the onset of covergence or divergence preceding the saccade coincides with the onset of preparation for the saccade.

In other words, it may be concluded that a change of points of fixation in space begins at once by two processes—convergence or divergence and the preparation of the program of the saccades. The fact that convergence or divergence begins before the eyes rotate towards the new object of fixation, and not after this rotation, appreciably shortens the time required for changing the points of fixation.

4. SCHEME OF EYE MOVEMENTS DURING CHANGE OF STATIONARY POINTS OF FIXATION IN SPACE

The study of many different records has shown that in any change of the points of fixation in space the process of convergence or di-

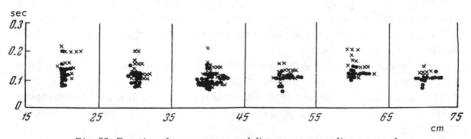

Fig. 92. Duration of convergence and divergence preceding a saccade.

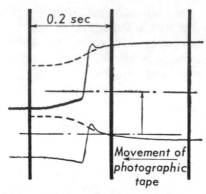

Fig. 93. Photokymographic record of eye movements during a change of stationary points of fixation in space. The broken lines are copies of the recording of divergence preceding the saccade, displaced by the magnitude of the saccade.

vergence is continuous, regardless of whether it is accompanied by saccades (when the points of fixation lie on different axes of the cyclopic eye) or not (when the points of fixation lie along the same axis of the cyclopic eye). In other words, the process of convergence or divergence of the eyes before, during, and after the saccade is the same process of continuous change in depth of the point of fixation. Any change of stationary points of fixation in space (unless these points are situated along the same axis of the cyclopic eye) consists of the sum of two independent eye movements—convergence or divergence, and saccade. When stationary points of fixation are situated on the same axis of the cyclopic eye, the eye movements during a change of these points may take place without a saccade.

A record of a change of the points of fixation in space (record made from both eyes on a slit photokymograph) is given in Fig. 93. The arrow shows the displacement of the axis of the cyclopic eye during the saccade. The broken lines are copies of the recording of the divergence preceding the saccade, displaced by the magnitude of the saccade. It is clear from the figure that the parts of the records of the divergence flow smoothly to make a single whole. The scheme illustrated in Fig. 94 can be constructed from the study of records such as these.

In the left part of the figure is shown a diagram of eye movements during a change from a point of fixation A to a more distant point of fixation B. In the right part is shown a diagram of the eye movements during a change from a point of fixation B to a point of fixation A nearer the subject.

The eye movements during a change from point of fixation A to point of fixation B are composed of: (a) divergence, preceding the saccade in the portion AC, during which the point of intersection of the optical axes moves along the axis of the cyclopic eye, directed to the point A; (b) saccades of the eyes, i.e., rotation of the axis of the cyclopic eye in the direction of point B and accompanied by continuing divergence; and (c) further divergence of the eyes, during which the point of intersection of the optical axes moves along the line DB, i.e., the axis of the cyclopic eye directed to the point B.

During the change from point of fixation B to point of fixation A, the movement of the eyes is composed of: (a) convergence preceding the saccade, during which the point of intersection of the optical axes moves along the line BE, i.e., along the axis of the cyclopic eye directed to point B; (b) saccades of the eyes, i.e., rotation of the axis of the cyclopic eye in the direction of point A, with continuing convergence; and (c) further convergence of the eyes, during which the point of intersection of the optical axes moves along FA, i.e., along the axis of the cyclopic eye directed to the point A. As we have said, sometimes a change of the points of fixation is accompanied by supplementary correcting saccades. In this case, the character of the eye movements remains as indicated in Fig. 94.

In many cases a very small corrective divergence or convergence is found at the end of the process of changing the points of fixation. This additional convergence or divergence introduces no essential change into the scheme of the eye movements, but leads to considerable scatter of the durations of convergence and divergence. A more complete idea of the character of the eye movements during changes of stationary points of fixation in space may be gained from study of Figs. 95, 96, and 97.

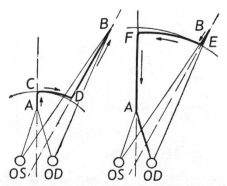

Fig. 94. Diagram of eye movements during a change of stationary points of fixation in space.

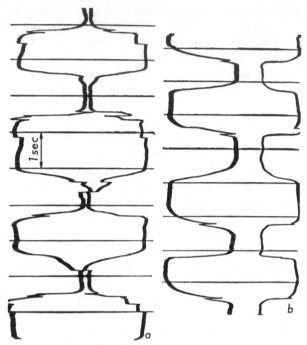

Fig. 95. Sample records of eye movements (photokymograph) during repeated replacement of one stationary fixed point by another.

5. APPARENT SIZE OF OBJECT AND DIRECTION OF GAZE

If the distance between the eyes and the object remains constant and only the apparent size is considered, the size of the object will depend primarily on the size of the retinal image and the position of

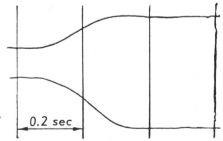

Fig. 96. Photokymographic record of eye movements during change of stationary points of fixation in space situated along the axis of the cyclopic eye.

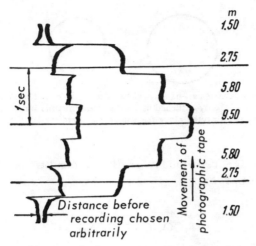

Fig. 97. Photokymographic record of eye movements during interchange of a series of stationary points of fixation in space.

the optical axes of the eyes. The tension of the muscles when the optical axes are in a certain position and the size of the retinal image are so related that, given the same retinal image with differences in convergence, the apparent size of the object will change, decreasing as the convergence increases. This relationship, arising as a result of our experiment, is responsible for the correct estimation of the size and position of an object in space (the decrease in the apparent size of an object as covergence increases, with a constant retinal image, can easily be determined on a Wheatstone stereoscope).

The system of the eye muscles is so constructed that, if there is no fixation (for example, in total darkness), when the eyes are rotated upward from a central position or downward, the axes of the eyes diverge slightly. This involuntary divergence of the optical axes places an additional load on the eye muscles during convergence. The additional load on the muscles, in cases when the eyes are strongly deviated from the central position upward or downward, naturally causes some decrease in the apparent size of the object. Special experiments have revealed the distortions arising in this case. The differences in apparent size of two equal circles (situated the same adequate distance from the observer's eyes) are shown in Fig. 98; the smaller circle corresponds to the position in which the eyes are turned upward to the limit, the larger, to the position in which the eyes are directed along the sagittal plane to the line of the horizon. Ordinarily, with relatively small rotations of the eyes, these distortions

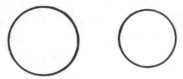

Fig. 98. Differences in the apparent size of two equal circles. The smaller circle corresponds to the position of the eyes turned upward to the limit; the larger circle corresponds to the position of the eyes directed along the sagittal plane to the horizon line.

can always be ignored (under ordinary conditions, they are never noticed by the observer).

CONCLUSIONS

Any change of stationary points of fixation in space is composed of two independent movements —convergence or divergence, and a saccade. The saccade is always preceded by an initial period of convergence or divergence. The duration of this period is approximately the same in all cases.

Chapter VI

EYE MOVEMENTS DURING PERCEPTION
OF MOVING OBJECTS

If a visual object is in movement, the observer's eyes usually move in pursuit of it. The aim of this pursuit is to make the retinal image of the object as stationary as necessary relative to the retina. By as stationary as necessary, we mean a velocity of movement of the retinal image so small that the eyes retain a high level of resolving power. The actual movement of pursuit is possible only if it is controlled by some form of system, hereinafter termed the system of pursuit.

If the movement of the visual test object is complex, the movements of the eyes will also be very complex. They may be composed of pursuit movements, saccades changing the points of fixation of the moving object, corrective saccades appearing under particularly complex conditions of perception, and, finally, movements of convergence and divergence of the optical axes, which may take place continuously as the need arises and are merged with the movement of pursuit.

1. INVOLUNTARY ASPECTS OF PURSUIT OF MOVING
OBJECTS

To determine to what extent the system of pursuit works involuntarily and automatically, a series of experiments was performed. In one experiment, P_2 caps were fixed to both anesthetized eyes of a subject, completely covering the cornea. The subject was in total darkness. Each cap was fitted with a small mirror. A beam of light was projected onto the mirror and reflected onto a screen as spots of light; by following these, the experimenter could estimate the movements of the subject's eyes and, if need be, record them.

When the subject was instructed to imagine that he was looking at an object, the character of the eye movements coincided with the character of the movements during the perception of stationary objects. A change in imaginary points of fixation situated in the sagittal plane at different distances from the eyes also was accompanied by a clearly defined convergence and divergence of the eyes. The only appreciable difference from normal was a decrease in the accuracy of fixation. Attempts to pursue the movement of the imaginary object smoothly did not have the desired result. Although it always appeared to the subject that the movements of his eyes were smooth and continuous, in fact they consisted entirely of separate fixations, saccades, convergences, and divergences.

In the next experiment, a smooth, uniformly illuminated screen was placed before the subject's open eyes. A P_1 cap was fixed to each eye. The records in this case showed that the subject could reproduce at will all types of eye movement except smooth movements of pursuit. An experiment described and illustrated earlier demonstrated that it was also impossible to obtain smooth pursuing movements when tracing the outline of a stationary figure with the eye. It may thus be concluded that in normal conditions the system of pursuit of the eyes cannot be operated at will without the presence of an object moving in the field of vision.

Usually we can start or stop completely at will the pursuit of an object moving in our field of vision. If the object is large enough, the system of pursuit is often set in motion involuntarily. Moreover, if the moving object occupies the whole field of vision or a large enough part of that field, in some conditions, once put into operation, the system of pursuit cannot be stopped until the object stops moving or the subject closes his eyes.

In one experiment the P_4 cap (see its description) was used. After the cap had been affixed to the eye, the subject saw objects only by means of the small mirror attached to the apparatus, i.e., by means of a mirror moving together with the eye. Under these conditions, eye movements evoked movements of the retinal image. The relationship between the angle of rotation of the eye and the angle of rotation of the retinal image was always very complex. The subject saw the objects clearly but could not choose his points of fixation at will, i.e., he could not use eye movements to obtain information on the spatial relationships between objects.

The fact that objects visible to the subject through the cap could not be examined at will created an unpleasant sensation for him. This unnatural state frequently had the result that the system of pursuit was set in operation involuntarily, and the eye began to make fruitless oscillatory searching movements, accompanied by oscillations of the visual images. In such conditions the subject could not stop his eye, i.e., he could not prevent his system of pursuit from functioning, and the oscillations of the eye continued until the end of the experiment.

If the image of an object moving with constant velocity appeared in the field of vision (in the mirror of the P_4 cap), this image was always pursued with acceleration. As soon as the eye began to follow the movement of the image of the object, the mirror of the cap turned also, and the apparent velocity of the moving image was increased (the velocity of the retinal image relative to the retina was increased). The eye, as it moved, made an appropriate correction, and this in turn led to a still greater increase in the apparent velocity. A series of these corrections accelerated the movement of the eye, and this acceleration continued as long as the visual image of the object remained within the field of vision. The subject's attempts to control their system of pursuit and make it more "intelligent" in these conditions likewise proved unsuccessful. Consequently, when the usual relationship between the movement of the eye and the displacement of the retinal image is disturbed, the system of pursuit cannot perform its function, although it tries to do so.

If a moving object is present in the field of vision, the observer can start and stop pursuit of the object at will. However, an observer can never (at least, without special training) interfere voluntarily with the actual process of pursuit and change its speed deliberately, making it greater or less than the speed of the moving object.

2. MINIMAL AND MAXIMAL VELOCITIES OF PURSUIT

We next attempted to determine the range within which the system of pursuit works if the object of perception moves at a uniform speed along a horizontal straight line lying in the frontal plane. For this purpose two series of experiments were carried out.

In most experiments, the movements of the visual test object were recorded at the same time as the eye movements. A spot of light from a slit source was divided into two parts so that one part, as an illuminated point, moved over a screen at which the subject looked, serving as the visual test object, while the other, in the form of a narrow vertical band, fell on the horizontal slit of a photokymograph and was used to record the movements of the object. From the beam of light reflected from the mirror affixed to the cap on the eye, which also fell on the slit of the photokymograph, the eye movements were recorded. Neither of the last two beams could be seen by the subject. Given the appropriate distances, the experimenter could always calculate the relationship between the recorded amplitudes of object movement and eye movement. From the simultaneous records of the movements of the eye and object, the experimenter could determine very accurately the degree to which the movements of the eye and of the object corresponded under different experimental conditions.

In the first series of experiments, the objects pursued by the subjects moved with a very low angular velocity. The records obtained showed that smooth pursuit begins when the speed of the object equals the speed of the irregular drift of the eye (always present during fixation). The smooth pursuing movement develops as a result of change of the irregular drift into a regular drift, i.e., a drift with a dominant direction. When the speed of the object is equal to one minute of arc per second, some degree of order can already be observed against the background of the drift, and this may be taken as smooth pursuit. When the speed of the object reaches 5 minutes of arc per second, the smooth pursuit is now perfectly clear, although the drift still causes marked distortion of this movement (Fig. 99). Not until the speed exceeds 10-15 minutes of arc per second is the drift hardly noticeable in the records. Pursuit of low velocity (measured in

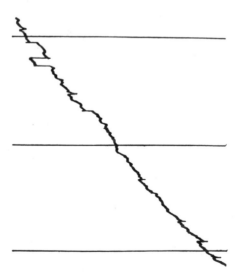

Fig. 99. Record of eye movements during pursuit of an object moving from left to right at a speed of 5 minutes of arc per second. The record clearly shows the drift of the eye and the small saccades.

units of minutes of arc per second) is usually accompanied by small involuntary saccades. The amplitude of these saccades and the frequency with which they appear differ only slightly from the amplitude and frequency of the saccades arising during fixation of a stationary object.

In the second series of experiments, the subjects pursued objects moving at high angular velocities. In this case, the ability to pursue was determined not only by the angular velocity with which the object moved, but also by whether this object had been present all the time in the subject's field of vision or had appeared unexpectedly and then rapidly disappeared from the visual field.

A certain period of time is required for pursuit to develop; if the moving object is present in the field of vision for less than this period (0.15 sec), pursuit is impossible. On the other hand, if the moving object remains in the field of vision, the conditions for pursuit become more favorable. The eye then has sufficient time to prepare for each individual pursuit or saccade, coinciding in direction with the moving object.

The saccadic movements serving to change the points of fixation last for hundredths of a second. During a saccade the eyes move in accordance with a definite law, and this movement differs sharply from the movement of pursuit. Nevertheless, saccades enable the details even of very fast moving objects to be examined, if they follow the direction in which the object is moving. In this case the object may attain a velocity of 400-500 deg/sec. Somewhat smaller velocities of movement of the object (350-400 deg/sec) may be accompanied by very brief movements of pursuit.

During free examination of stationary objects, the duration of the shortest, and at the same time the commonest, fixations lies within 0.20 and 0.25 sec. This duration of fixation evidently corresponds to satisfactory conditions of perception. There is therefore reason to believe that satisfactory conditions for perception of moving objects arise if pursuit movements of a duration of 0.20-0.25 sec become possible. When a moving object is seen continuously, as the experiments show, such satisfactory conditions of perception are possible if the speed of the object does not exceed 200 deg/sec. If the object appears every time unexpectedly, such conditions arise only at speeds of 150-100 deg/sec.

Although we have considered eye movements only, it must be remembered that under ordinary conditions of pursuit of moving objects the observer's head also turns and that this essentially facilitates his task.

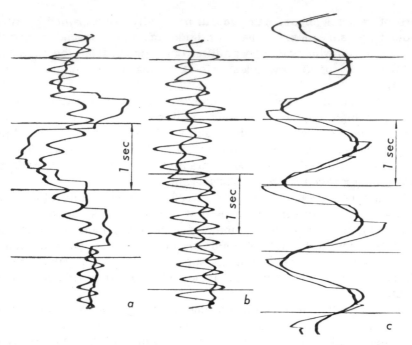

Fig. 100. Sample simultaneous records of movements of the object and eye. Smooth lines—movements of the object. Movements of the eyes are characterized by corrective saccades: a) unsuccessful attempt at pursuing; b) shift in phase clearly seen on the record (the result of delay of the eye), amplitude of the oscillations of the eye diminished by comparison with the movement of the object; c) more accurate pursuit.

3. EYE MOVEMENTS DURING PURSUIT IN COMPLEX CONDITIONS

In many experiments the object moved with an acceleration which was a complex function of time. Here, the records clearly showed how the system of pursuit works and what its possibilities are under conditions of varying complexity.

The records shown in Fig. 100 will perhaps give some idea of the system of pursuit under complex conditions.

It will be noted that during the attempt to pursue the object, the observer's eyes attempt to repeat the movement of the object, but do so only after a slight delay (0.1-0.2 sec). This delay can easily be detected from the shifts in phase on some of the records in Fig. 100, which reflect attempts made by the eye to follow the oscillating movements of the object. When trying to follow the movements of the object, the system of pursuit continually introduces corrections, as shown by the fact that when the oscillations of the object are of high frequency, the amplitude of the oscillations of the eye may be considerably less than the amplitude of oscillations of the object (Fig. 100). This is because before one movement can be completed, the eye begins to take part in a second movement, following the object. The attempt of the eyes to pursue the object is often accompanied by corrective saccades, as a result of which the retinal image of the object falls on the fovea.

It may be concluded from a study of these records that the eye obtains the information essential for pursuit in two states—a state of fixation and a state of pursuit. In the first case, the essential information is given by evaluation of the angular velocity of movement of the object, and in the second by evaluation of the difference between the angular velocities of the object and the moving eye. The information thus gained may be used in two ways. Sometimes the eye changes

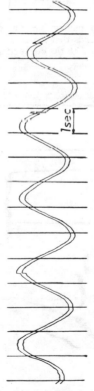

Fig. 101. Movement of both eyes recorded during pursuit of a pendulum oscillating in the frontal plane.

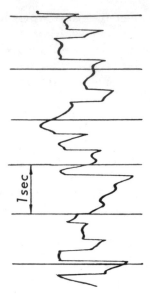

Fig. 102. Eye movements recorded during pursuit of an object taking part in a complex movement. It is clear from the records that the sharp change in the velocity and direction of movement of the eye is coordinated with the correcting saccade.

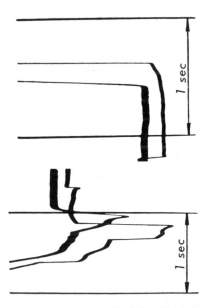

Fig. 103. Records of movements of an object (thick lines) and the eye, showing clearly the delay in the movements of the eye initiated during pursuit.

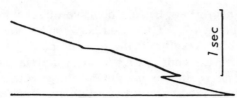

Fig. 104. Record of movements of the eye during pursuit of an object moving at uniform velocity, and appearing unexpectedly in the right peripheral part of the subject's field of vision. Pursuit at the necessary speed begins instantaneously following a saccade.

its velocity smoothly (in magnitude and direction), following the move-ment of the object (Fig. 101). Sometimes, however, it begins to move at once at a certain velocity or sharply changes its velocity (in magnitude and direction). This second case is always preceded by a saccade, after which a movement follows immediately (within millisec-onds) at a velocity equal to or close to the velocity of the object. In other words, the sharp change in velocity is always timed to take place during the correcting saccade (Fig. 102).

If a moving object appears suddenly in the foveal region of the subject's field of vision, naturally pursuit cannot begin instantaneously. For pursuit to begin, some time is required for the system of pursuit to become operative; the records show this time to be approximately 0.1-0.2 sec, usually 0.15-0.17 sec (Fig. 103). If the moving object appears suddenly and the subject sees it with the peripheral part of the retina, preparation for pursuit (requiring 0.1 0.2 sec) takes place on the basis of data obtained from the periphery, and is accompanied by simultaneous preparation for a saccade to the object. It is most important that the saccade always take place after the preparation for pursuit, i.e., when the system of pursuit "knows" approximately with what angular velocity it must carry out its pursuing function. For this reason, after the saccade has taken place and the image of the object lies in the central part of the retina, pursuit begins practically instantaneously, within milliseconds (Fig. 104).

Records such as those in Figs. 102 and 104 suggest that the system of pursuit is prepared for its pursuing function or for a sharp change in its velocity and direction not after but before the saccade, i.e., during the fixation preceding the saccade, or during the pursuit preceding the saccade. Experiments show that participation of the eyes in the process of pursuit begins not at the end of the saccade, but at its beginning. In other words, the instructions to begin the saccade and the new act of pursuit take place simultaneously or almost simul-taneously. Since the velocity of the saccade is large (and its duration small), displacement of the eyes resulting from premature pursuit may be taken as negligible, but the positive effect is substantial, and there is no pause in the work of the eyes between the end of the saccade and the beginning of pursuit. If the eyes do not begin their pursuing function until after a saccade, as a result of inertia they would not be able to begin pursuit quite so instantaneously (within milliseconds). If a moving object pursued by an observer disappears unexpectedly and instantaneously, the eyes cease their pursuit, slow down gradually, and eventually stop completely (after approximately 0.1 second).

4. PURSUIT ACCOMPANIED BY CONVERGENCE AND DIVERGENCE OF THE OPTICAL AXES

When an object of perception, moving in space, moves nearer to or further from the observer, pursuit is accompanied by convergence or divergence of the optical axes and is the most complex case of eye movement.

I mentioned earlier that the pursuing movement of the eyes and convergence or divergence of the optical axes, although different types of movements, take place in such close cooperation during pursuit that they cannot be differentiated on records. This merger is evidently explained by the fact that convergence and divergence have much in common with pursuit and may, in some cases, completely take over its function. For example, if a moving object shifts along the axis of the

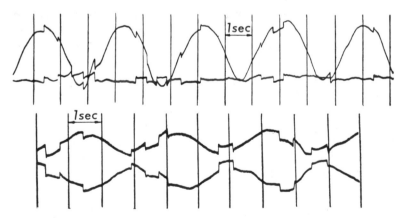

Fig. 105. Records of eye movements during pursuit of a pendulum oscillating in the sagittal plane passing through the right eye (top figure) and between the eyes (bottom figure).

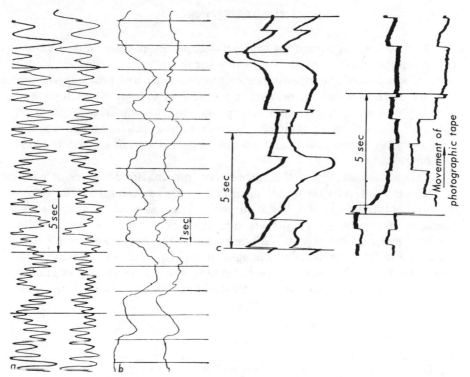

Fig. 106. Records of eye movements during pursuit of objects accompanied by complex movements. a) Oscillations, b) irregular movement in space, c) during perception of stereo-scopic picture.

cyclopic eye, pursuit is reduced to movements of convergence or divergence and correcting saccades.

It may thus be considered that the convergence or divergence of the optical axes is a movement during which the point of fixation slides along the axis of the cyclopic eye. The intersection of the optical axes may be displaced (as a result of convergence or divergence) along the axis of the cyclopic eye relatively quickly and suddenly during a change of stationary or moving points of fixation, or, on the other hand, steadily and slowly during pursuit of a moving object. The axis of the cyclopic eye may itself be displaced in space, making steady rotations during pursuit and sudden movement during saccades.

Sample records of eye movements when the object of perception performs complex movements in space are shown in Figs. 105 and 106. These records demonstrate to some extent the possibilities open to the system of pursuit and the system of the eye muscles.

CONCLUSIONS

The system of pursuit of the eyes cannot be put into action voluntarily, in the absence of an object moving in the field of vision. Under
normal conditions, no smooth pursuit movements are possible without
the presence of an object moving in the field of vision. Smooth pursuit
can begin when objects move at speeds equal to those of the drift of
the eye arising during fixation. Satisfactory conditions of perception
are possible when the speed of the object does not exceed 100–200
deg/sec.

The eye must obtain the necessary information for pursuit while
in the state of fixation or in the state of steady pursuit. The information obtained can be used in two ways. In some cases, the eye
changes its speed (in magnitude and direction) steadily, and follows
the movement of the object. In other cases, the eye begins to move at
once at a definite velocity or changes its speed suddenly (in magnitude
and direction). In these circumstances, the instantaneous beginning
or sudden change in velocity is coordinated with a saccade of the eyes.

Chapter VII

EYE MOVEMENTS DURING PERCEPTION
OF COMPLEX OBJECTS

In this chapter we shall try to determine how the human eye examines complex objects and what principles govern this process. For example, it may seen to some people that when we examine an object we must trace its outlines with our eye and, by analogy with tactile sensation, "palpate" the object. Others may consider that, when looking at a picture, we scan the whole of its surface more or less uniformly with our eyes.

The problem of eye movements during perception of pictures during reading, during the perception of optical illusions, and during comparison of distances is investigated below. To round out our study of the role of eye movements, we shall also consider the question of perception during which the subject cannot voluntarily use his eye movements or choose points of fixation.

1. EYE MOVEMENTS DURING PERCEPTION OF COMPLEX
OBJECTS

Before reading the text, the reader should quickly look over the records of eye movements shown in Figs. 107-124. Study of such records as these suggests first of all that, when examining complex objects, the human eye fixates mainly on certain elements of these objects. Any picture (unless it is a uniform background or a repetitive mosaic) contains different elements; the eye rests much longer on some of these than on others, while some elements may receive little or no attention. What distinguishes the elements particularly attracting the observer's attention, and what are the characteristic features of those elements which do not draw his attention ?

Analysis of the eye-movement records shows that the elements attracting attention contain, in the observer's opinion, may contain,

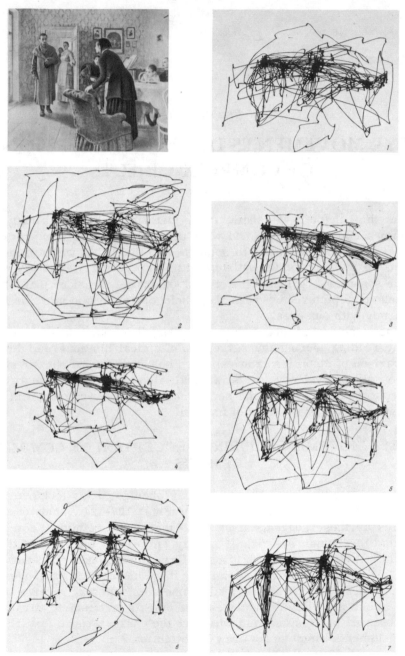

Fig. 107. Reproduction from I. E. Repin's picture "An Unexpected Visitor" and records of the eye movements of seven different subjects. Each subject examined the picture freely (without instruction) with both eyes for 3 minutes.

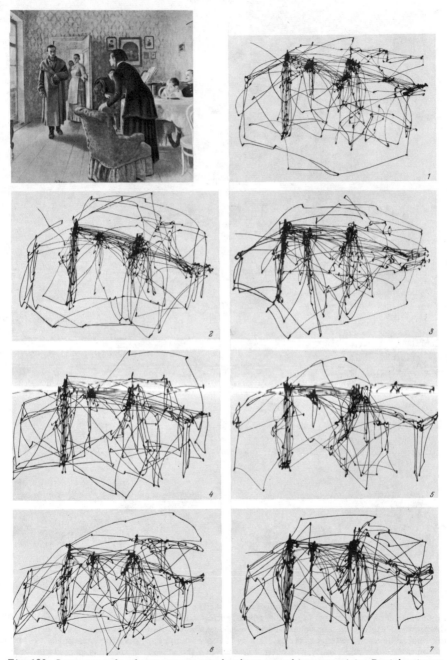

Fig. 108. Seven records of eye movements by the same subject, examining Repin's picture freely with both eyes. The records, arranged in chronological order, lasted 3 minutes. The interval between records was 1 or 2 days.

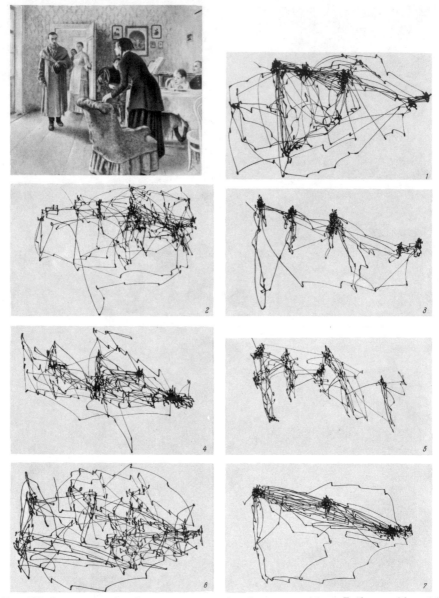

Fig. 109. Seven records of eye movements by the same subject. Each record lasted 3 minutes. The subject examined the reproduction with both eyes. 1) Free examination of the picture. Before the subsequent recording sessions, the subject was asked to: 2) estimate the material circumstances of the family in the picture; 3) give the ages of the people; 4) surmise what the family had been doing before the arrival of the "unexpected visitor"; 5) remember the clothes worn by the people; 6) remember the position of the people and objects in the room; 7) estimate how long the "unexpected visitor" had been away from the family.

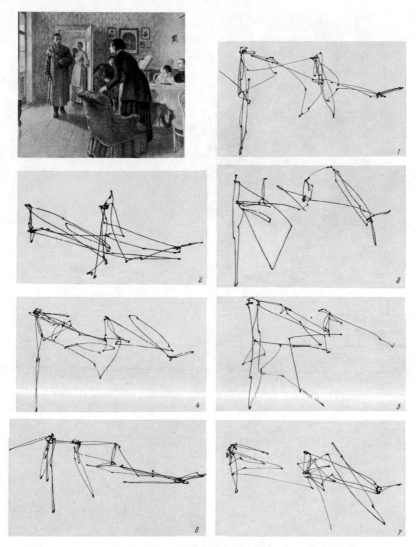

Fig. 110. Record of the eye movements for 3 minutes during free examination, divided into seven consecutive parts. The duration of each part is about 25 seconds.

information useful and essential for perception. Elements on which the eye does not fixate, either in fact or in the observer's opinion, do not contain such information.

Let us now try to explain and prove this statement. First we will note that special attention or indifference to the elements of a picture is in no way due to the number of details composing the elements.

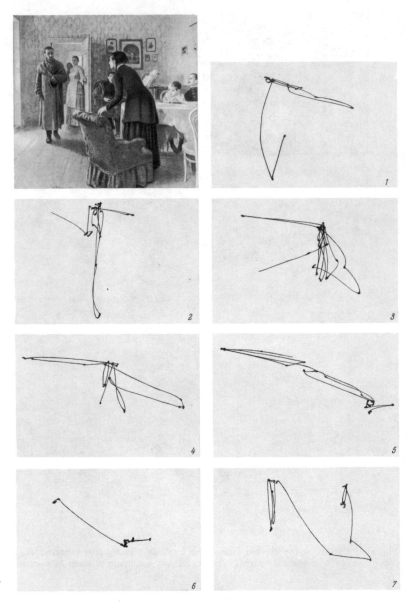

Fig. 111

Fig. 111 is a record of the eye movements for 35 seconds during free examination. The recording is divided into seven consecutive parts of 5 seconds each. The number of fixations in each part of the record is: 1, 18; 2, 16; 3, 18; 4, 14; 5, 17; 6, 13; and 7, 15. In Fig. 112 each point of fixation of the eye movements illustrated in Fig. 111 is covered with a black circle. The size of the circles corresponds to the size of the central fovea of the subject's eye (1.3°). This figure shows which elements of the reproduction were fixated by the central fovea and in what order during examination of the picture for 35 seconds.

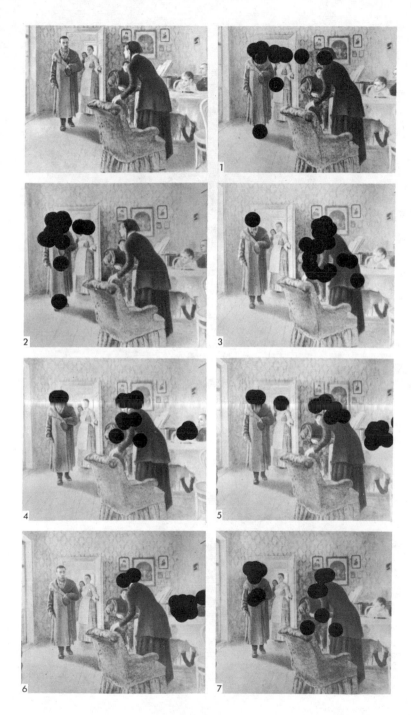

Fig. 112

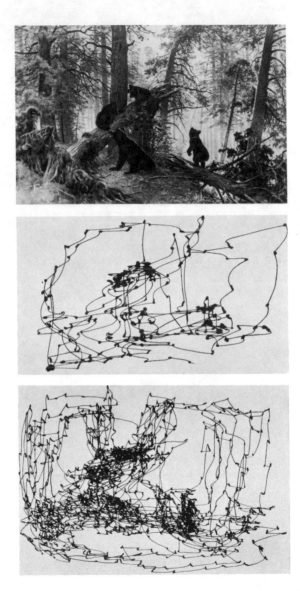

Fig. 113. Reproduction of I. I. Shishkin's picture "Morning in the Pine Forest." The records of the eye movements were made during free examination of the picture with both eyes for 2 and 30 minutes.

For example, the figure of the hunter in Fig. 118 particularly attracts the observer's attention although it is no more detailed than many other elements of the picture. Although the bears in Fig. 113 have fewer details than the branches of the trees, they attract most attention. It is clear from the records of Fig. 117 that the eye fixates mainly along the line of the horizon and on the trunk of the birch trees, although in this picture the details composing the grass and leaves are especially

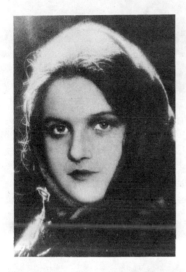

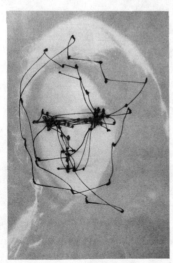

Fig 114. Photograph of a girl's face. Record of the eye movements during free examination of the photograph with both eyes for one minute.

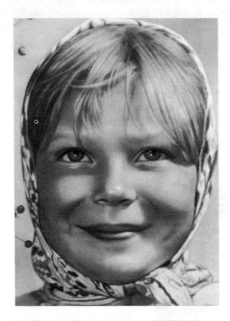

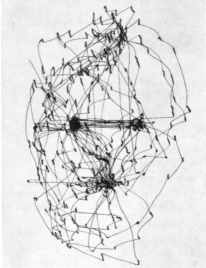

Fig. 115. The first page of the magazine "Ogonek," No. 23 (1959): "Girl from the Volga" (photograph by S. Fridlyand). Record of the eye movements during free examination of the photograph with both eyes for 3 minutes.

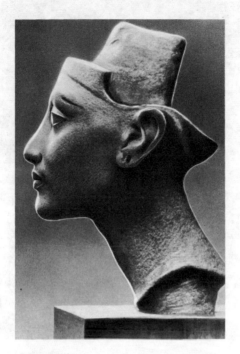

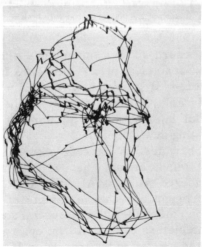

Fig. 116. Head of the Egyptian Queen Nefertiti (16th century B.C.). Record of eye movements during free examination of a photograph of the sculptured head with both eyes for 2 minutes.

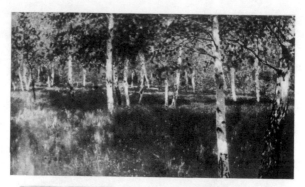

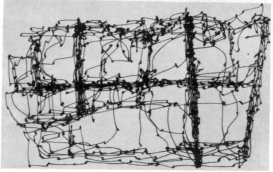

Fig. 117. Reproduction of I. I. Levitan's picture "The Birch Wood." Record of eye movements during free examination of the reproduction with both eyes for 10 minutes.

numerous. Any record of eye movements shows that, per se, the number of details contained in an element of the picture does not determine the degree of attention attracted to this element. This is easily understandable, for in any picture, the observer can obtain essential and useful information by glancing at some details, while others tell him nothing new or useful.

Similarly, the brightest or darkest elements of a picture are not necessarily those which attract the eye (if the brightness of these elements is considered alone). All records of the eye movements show that nèither bright nor dark elements of a picture attract the observer's attention unless they give essential and useful information. For example, in the picture in Fig. 113 the eye rests most on the dark brown figures of the bears; in the picture in Fig. 117 the observer's attention is attracted by the white trunks of the birch trees; in Fig. 118, by the figure of the hunter which is almost completely merged with the background; and so on.

For many observers one color is more pleasing than another, and
sometimes the expression "my favorite color" is heard. Most of the
reproductions used in my experiments for free examination by the
subjects were colored. Sometimes both colored and black-and-white
reproductions of the same size taken from the same picture were used.
However, in no case did the corresponding records reveal any appreciable influence of color on the distribution of the points of fixation.
It must be concluded that if the color of an element has no special
significance and is irrelevant to the meaning of the picture under
examination, it will have no effect on the character of the eye movements. The results described in Chapter II show that an important role
in the process of vision is played by the outlines of objects perceived.
The question arises: to what extent does this importance of outline

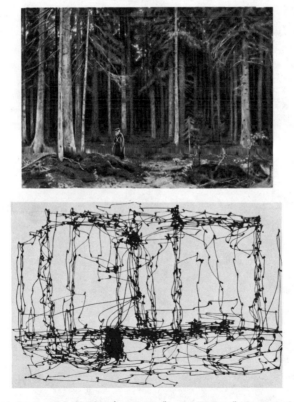

Fig. 118. Reproduction of I.I. Shishkin's picture "In the Forest." Record of the movements
of one eye during free examination of the picture with both eyes for 10 minutes.

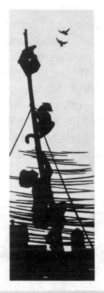

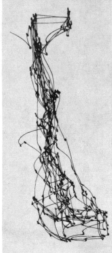

Fig. 119. Drawing by V. Surkov. Record of the movements of one eye during free examination of picture with both eyes for 3 minutes.

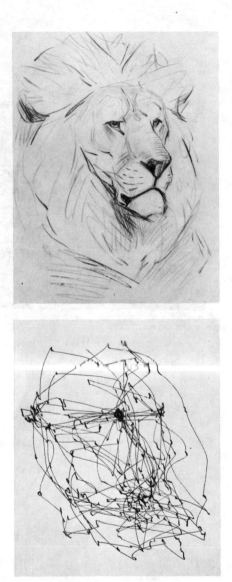

Fig. 120. Drawing by V. A. Vatagin. Record of the movements of one eye during free examination of the picture with both eyes for 2 minutes.

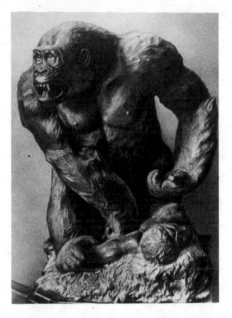

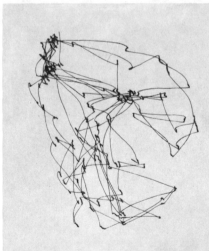

Fig. 121. V.A. Vatagin's sculpture "Gorilla." Record of the movements of one eye during free examination of a photograph of the sculpture by both eyes for one minute.

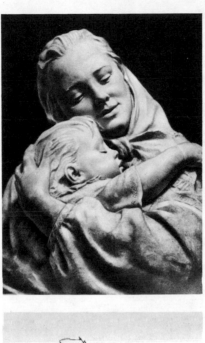

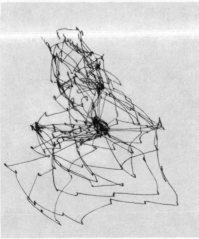

Fig. 122. G.L. Petrushavich's sculpture "My Child." Record of the movements of one eye during free examination of a photograph of the sculpture with both eyes for 2 minutes.

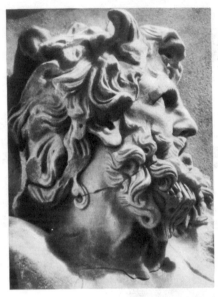

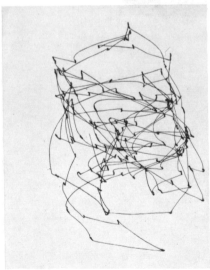

Fig. 123. Photograph of the frieze from the Pergamon altar. Head of Clitus. Record of the movements of one eye during free examination of the photograph with both eyes for one minute.

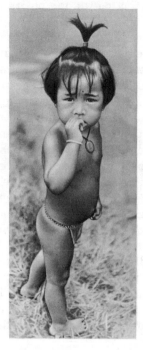

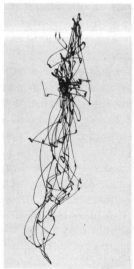

Fig. 124. "Ogonek," No. 21 (1959): photograph of a girl by S. Orlina. Record of the movements of one eye during free examination of the photograph with both eyes for one minute.

influence the eye movements and the distribution of the points of fixation?

Analysis of Figs. 107-124 shows that the outlines themselves have no effect on the character of the eye movements. In the movements of the eye we have no analogy with the movements of the hand of a blind person, tracing the outlines and contours. Outlines and contours are important for the appearance of the visual image, but when the image has appeared and is seen constinously, the observer has no need to concern himself specially with borders and contours. Borders and contours are only elements from which, together with other no less important elements, our perception is composed and the object recognized. Clearly the outlines of an object will attract an observer's attention if the actual shape of the outline includes important and essential information. For example, when examining the sculpture of Queen Nefertiti's head (Fig. 116), the observer directs nearly all his attention to the profile of the head, to the outline of the sculpture. It is easy to see that the main features of the sculpture are concentrated in these places, thus enabling the observer to form a complete representation of the head. On the other hand, the record in Fig. 119 which shows the eye movements during free examination of a picture that is purely in silhouette is completely indistinguishable from the record of ordinary pictures.

All the records given in this chapter, as well as others not mentioned here, show conclusively that the character of the eye movements is either completely independent of or only very slightly dependent on the material of the picture and how it was made, provided that it is flat or nearly flat. Examination of objects situated in a room or examination of a sculptured head in which a change is made from points of fixation situated at different distances from the observer is accompanied by convergence and divergence of the optical axes, and differs from the perception of flat objects only in this new type of movement (i.e., convergence of the eyes).

Records of eye movements show that the observer's attention is usually held only by certain elements of the picture. As already noted, the study of these elements shows that they give information allowing the meaning of the picture to be obtained. Eye movements reflect the human thought processes; so the observer's thought may be followed to some extent from records of eye movements (the thought accompanying the examination of the particular object). It is easy to determine from these records which elements attract the observer's eye (and, consequently, his thought), in what order, and how often.

If we look at the records in Figs. 107 and 108, made during free examination of Repin's picture "An Unexpected Visitor," we can see that in all 14 records the faces of the people shown in the picture attract the observers' attention much more than the figures, and the figures more than the objects in the room, and so on. Moreover, even the faces of the different people attract attention unequally, depending on the place they occupy in the theme of the picture.

When looking at a human face, an observer usually pays most attention to the eyes, the lips, and the nose. The other parts of the face are given much more cursory consideration. Looking at the record in Fig. 114, we see that in this portrait attention is drawn almost exclusively to the girl's beautiful expressive eyes. The observer pays much less attention to the lips and nose. In the photograph of the smiling girl in Fig. 115, the lips attract far more attention; the reason for this will be clear to the reader when he looks at the photograph. It is curious that, when examining the picture of the lion's head (Fig. 120) and the sculpture of a gorilla (Fig. 121), most of the points of fixation of attention are found on the eyes, nose, and mouth of the animals.

The human eyes and lips (and the eyes and mouth of an animal) are the most mobile and expressive elements of the face. The eyes and lips can tell an observer the mood of a person and his attitude towards the observer, the steps he may take next moment, and so on. It is therefore absolutely natural and understandable that the eyes and lips attract the attention more than any other part of the human face.

During the examination of the photograph of a sculpture (Fig. 122) the observer pays special attention to the face of the sleeping child (the closed eyes, lips, nose), the mother's smiling face (the lips attract special attention), and the mother's hand holding the child's head. It is easy to see that the child's face reflects blissful sleep and the mother's face and her tender smile express the happiness of motherhood, while the mother's hand expresses care and affection. In this case, then, the observer fixated on the elements which revealed to him the main theme of this picture.

The observer's attention is frequently drawn to elements which do not give important information but which, in his opinion, may do so. Often an observer will focus his attention on elements that are unusual in the particular circumstances, unfamiliar, incomprehensible, and so on. For example, many of the points of fixation in the recordings in Figs. 117 and 118 fall on the horizon line. Evidently the observer was examining the horizon in the hope of finding something important. In

Fig. 118 he was interested in the gap between the trees. In Fig. 124 he spent considerable time examining the amusing tuft of hair on the child's head, and so on. A careful examination of the two series of records in Figs. 107 and 108 showed, that despite the great similarity among all 14 records, the similarity is greater in the seven records of Fig. 108, which reflect the process of perception and thought of a single observer, than in the seven records of Fig. 107, which were obtained from seven different observers. It may be concluded that individual observers differ in the way they think and, therefore, differ also to some extent in the way they look at things.

All the observers whose eye movements are shown in Figs. 107 and 108 were well educated people and were well acquainted with Repin's picture. This evidently accounts for the generally considerable similarity between all the records. Perhaps the records would have been much less similar if the observers had differed more in cultural level and education. Undoubtedly, observers familiar both with the picture and the epoch represented in it would examine the picture differently from people seeing it for the first time and unfamiliar with the epoch it represents.

In just the same way it would be natural to assume that a complex object of perception understood by a physicist but unfamiliar to a biologist (or vice versa) will be examined quite differently by a physicist and a biologist.

Depending on the task in which a person is engaged, i.e., depending on the character of the information which he must obtain, the distribution of the points of fixation on an object will vary correspondingly, because different items of information are usually localized in different parts of an object. This is confirmed by Fig. 109. This figure shows that, depending on the task facing the subject, the eye movements varied. For example, in response to the instruction "estimate the material circumstances of the family shown in the picture," the observer paid particular attention to the women's clothing and the furniture (the armchair, stool, tablechloth, and so on). In response to the instruction " give the ages of the people shown in the picture," all attention was concentrated on their faces. In response to the instruction "surmise what the family was doing before the arrival of the 'unexpected visitor,'" the observer directed his attention particularly to the objects arranged on the table, the girl's and the woman's hands, and to the music. After the instruction "remember the clothes worn by the people in the picture," their clothing was examined. The instruction "remember the position of the people and objects in the room," caused the observer to examine the whole room and all the objects. His attention was even drawn to the chair leg shown in the left part of the picture which he had hitherto not observed. Finally, the instruction "estimate how long the 'unexpected visitor' had been away from the family," caused the observer to make particularly intensive movements of the eyes between the faces of the children and the face of the person entering the room. In this case he was undoubtedly trying to find the answer by studying the expressions on the faces and trying to determine whether the children recognized the visitor or not.

Records of the eye movements after an instruction are interesting because they help in the analysis of the significance of eye movements during the free examination of a picture; they show clearly that the importance of the elements giving information is determined by the problem facing the observer, and that this importance may vary within extremely wide limits.

It is clear from Figs. 107 and 108 that the observer's attention rested on the faces and figures depending on their significance for the picture as a whole. It should be noted that the scale of the figures and objects and their position in the picture—in other words, everything which we call the composition of the picture—also has definite importance. The figure of the woman, being the largest and being centrally situated, attracts more attention than any of the other figures. Hence composition is the means whereby the artist to some extent may compel the viewer to perceive what is portrayed in the picture.

If the eye movements are recorded for several minutes during perception of an object, the record obtained will clearly show that, when changing its points of fixation, the observer's eye repeatedly returns to the same elements of the picture. Additional time spent on perception is not used to examine the secondary elements, but to reexamine the most important elements. The impression is created that the perception of a picture is usually composed of a series of "cycles," each of which has much in common. For example, it is clear from Fig. 114 that the examination of the portrait in fact was reduced to the repeated alternate fixation on first one and then the other of the girl's eyes. The same can be seen in Fig. 115. The records in Fig. 113, one of which continued for 2 minutes, and the other for 10 minutes, generally speaking, differ only very slightly. The distribution of the points of fixation and the character of the eye movements were almost identical. It should be noted here that, although the records were obtained from the same observer, the interval between the experiments was a whole month. The reiterative movements of the eyes are seen particularly well in Fig. 116. In the 2 minutes, the observer cast his eyes several times around the profile of the sculptured head.

Analysis of these complex records of eye movements shows that the duration of a cycle during which the observer's eye can cover the whole picture amounts sometimes to several seconds, sometimes to several tens of seconds. The more complex an object and the more associations it arouses, the longer the duration of this cycle.

A reproduction of Repin's picture "An Unexpected Visitor" is shown in Fig. 110 with a 3-minute record of the eye movements during free examination of the picture by an observer. The record as a whole has been divided into seven consecutive parts, the duration of each part being 25 sec (during the experiment the sheet of photosensitive paper on which the record was made was changed very quickly every 25 sec). Analysis of these separate records shows that each of them, roughly speaking, corresponds to a cycle during which the eye stops and examines the most important elements of the picture. In each part, the observer's eye examines the faces of all the people shown in the picture.   In other words, during a 3-minute examination of the picture, the observer directed his attention at least seven different times to each face.

The records in Fig. 109 show that this cyclical pattern in the examination of pictures is dependent not only on what is shown on the picture, but also on the problem facing the observer and the information that he hopes to gain from the picture. For example, the record made following the instruction "estimate the ages of the people shown in the picture" shows relatively few reiterated movements.   After the instruction "estimate how long the unexpected visitor has been away from the family," there were several times more reiterated movements.

This cyclical pattern followed in the examination of objects evidently reflects some special features of our perception and thought. In this connection I shall do no more than mention the purely conjectural hypotheses which have been put forward.

In order to observe the special features of the eye movements in the initial stage of examination of Repin's familiar picture "An Unexpected Visitor," an interrupted 35-second record was made of the eye movements of an observer freely examining the picture. The record of the eye movements as a whole was divided into seven consecutive records, each 5 seconds long (the sheets of photosensitive paper were again changed quickly, every 5 seconds in this experiment). The results are shown in Figs. 111 and 112. In Fig. 112 all the points of fixation of the observer's attention were superposed on the picture and covered with black circles. The circles corresponded in size to the angular magnitude of the central fovea of the observer's eye (1.3°). In other words, the circles may be regarded as the projection of the central fovea of the observer's eye onto the picture in the conditions of this particular experiment.

Analysis of the experimental results is facilitated by Fig. 112. This figure shows that during the first 5 seconds the observer examined the man entering the room. The observer's attention was focused mainly on the man's face and the upper part of his body. By the end of this period, the observer had examined the visitor's boots and the faces of the women standing by the open door. Altogether, during this first 5-second period, the observer changed points of fixation 18 times. Apparently 16 of the fixations enabled the observer to gain at least a general impression of the identity of the "unexpected" person. Two fixations only were devoted to the study of the faces of the women standing by the open door (secondary characters). In the second 5-second period, the points of fixation were mainly situated along the line of sight of the man entering the room (directed at the face of the elderly woman) and along the line of sight of the woman (directed at the man's face). During this period, the observer was apparently investigating the relationship between the two main characters in the picture. It is possible that during this period the observer also to some extent formed a clear idea of the main theme of the picture. During this second 5-second period, the observer changed points of fixation 16 times. The third 5-second period was mainly devoted to the study of the elderly woman (her face and figure) and of the woman sitting by the piano. Characteristically, this study, like the preceding periods, was accompanied by fixation on the face of the man entering the room. The third period included 18 fixations. During the fourth 5-second period, the observer continued to study the main characters and began to examine the faces of the children sitting by the table. The fourth 5-second period included 14 fixations. During the fifth 5-second period, all the active characters were examined, but the main attention was given to the children. The fifth period included 17 fixations. Apparently, the fifth period concluded the first cycle of examination of the picture; the eye movements in the sixth and seventh periods largely repeated those made in the previous periods.

The results of the experiment illustrated in Figs. 111 and 112 suggest that the observer's eye examined all the more important elements of the picture during the first 25 seconds, and the observer himself evidently obtained a general idea of the theme of the picture.

Characteristically, during each 5-second period the observer directed his attention at least once to the man entering the room. During perception of the picture, the observer's thought was constantly directed to the "unexpected visitor," with which figure all the remaining elements of the picture were linked and compared. In the course of 25 seconds, the observer changed points of fixation 83 times (an average of more than three points of fixation per second). The number of points of fixation, and their distribution in space and time give the reader some idea of the perception of so complex an object as the picture "An Unexpected Visitor."

In conclusion, I must stress once again that the distribution of the points of fixation on an object, the order in which the observer's attention moves from one point of fixation to another, the duration of the fixations, the distinctive cyclic pattern of examination, and so on are determined by the nature of the object and the problem facing the observer at the moment of perception.

The material in this section clearly can be regarded as merely the beginning of the study of the perception of complex objects by recording the eye movements.

The many pictures included in this section should be regarded by the interested reader not merely as an illustration to the written text, but also as material for study. I hope that some of these pictures will be used by other authors. On many records taken from these pictures we can see that during perception many of the elements of the picture are not perceived by foveal vision. This is illustrated particularly clearly in Fig. 112. Foveal vision is reserved mainly for those elements containing essential information needed by the observer during perception.

In this connection, we cannot help thinking how important and biologically desirable is this heterogeneous structure of the retina, particularly, the fact that a fovea is present. By means of the fovea centralis, man sees many details only around the point of fixation, i.e., around a point which, as a rule, provides essential information. The lower resolving power of the eye periphery is useful because it enables less essential information to be obtained and facilitates the differentiation between the useful and useless information.

2. EYE MOVEMENTS IN READING

The first studies of eye movements in reading were evidently made by Javal (1879). His results were obtained by visual observation of the

subject's eyes.   The first photographic record of eye movements
during reading was obtained by Dodge in 1899 (see Taylor, 1957).
Several other authors have subsequently studied this problem (Buswell,
1937; Gilbert, 1953; Taylor, 1957).   Since I have not personally made
any detailed study of eye movements during reading, the data given
in this section are mainly compiled from other sources.

Some idea of the eye movements during reading is given by the
record in Fig. 125, made by means of the P_1 cap.   The subject in this

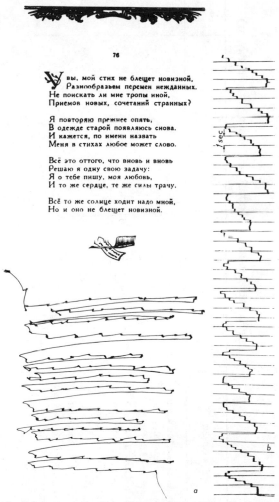

Fig. 125. Record of the eye movements of a subject reading a Shakespeare sonnet. Record
on stationary photosensitive paper (a) and on moving phototape of a photokymograph (b).

Table 2. Assessment of Skill in Reading (after Taylor)

Grades	1	2	3	4	5	6	Grade school	High school	College
Fixations per 100 words	240	200	170	136	118	105	95	83	75
Retraces per 100 words	55	45	37	30	26	23	18	15	11
Mean range of recognition during fixation of words	0.42	0.50	0.59	0.73	0.85	0.95	1.05	1.21	1.33
Mean duration of fixation (sec)	0.33	0.30	0.26	0.24	0.24	0.24	0.24	0.24	0.23
Mean rate of understanding (number of words per minute)	75	100	138	180	216	233	255	296	340

experiment was a student with average reading ability. One of the records was made on stationary photographic paper, the other by means of a photokymograph on moving oscillographic paper.

Examination of the second record shows clearly that during reading the duration of the fixations usually lies between 0.2 and 0.4 sec, with a mean value of 0.3 sec for this particular subject. During reading the character of the eye movements remains the same as during examination of other stationary objects if the natural regularity and succession of the eye movement along the lines of the text are now counted. The same record also shows that the reading of each line ends with a prolonged fixation (or two fixations), almost a whole second in duration. These prolonged fixations correspond to the long process of analysis of what has been read, in this case the line of the poem. Prolonged fixations are found during the reading of any text; the more complicated the text and the more numerous the thoughts, associations, and ideas evoked by the word or line read, the longer the fixation. These results indicate that the required resolving power of a printed text is maintained entirely by the foveal and parafoveal region of the retina.

A detailed study of the eye movements during reading, with a large number of students used as subjects, yielded results which, when presented as a table, could be used to evaluate methods of teaching pupils in various grades to read.

Records of the eye movements of 5000 students were used by Taylor to compile this table (Table 2). The table gives the mean values of the elements constituting the art of reading, which can be studied by suitable experimental techniques. The mean range of recognition per fixation by the children studying in the first six grades was less than one word (if a word is regarded as consisting of ten printed symbols). The mean range of recognition per fixation by the college students was 1.33 words. It was found that students trained by means of special tachistoscopes have an increased range of recognition per fixation, although no significant changes were observed in reading speed. As the students continued to develop, the number of fixations (per 100 words of text) fell to one-third the original number, while the number of retraces during reading fell to one-fifth. The duration of the fixation showed little change and in general remained the same as during free examination of any stationary object. The rate of understanding (the number of recognized words per minute) increased fourfold.

Investigations have shown that a person who reads aloud badly usually looks at a word when pronouncing it and, in doing so, makes two or more fixational pauses. Such a person does not run ahead of the word being pronounced with his eyes. A person who reads aloud fluently does not dwell on the word being pronounced, sometimes running along the line with his eyes for several words in advance.

Although some people can be taught to read at a speed of 1000 or more words per minute, the average reader cannot attain such a result even with training. Usually people who can be taught to read very quickly read very quickly before training. There is a considerable individual scatter in relation to speed of reading. Records have shown that teachers usually read at a speed of 350-500 words per minute, i.e., that most of them do not read better than students in Grade 9. Most adults read at a speed less than 300 words per minute. Many students read at the same speed as grade school pupils.

In 1935, Taylor examined a student who was a very fast reader. He read at the speed of between 600 and 2200 words per minute. When reading at speeds of between 1000 and 1500 words per minute, he could recite word for word extracts from high-school textbooks. When reading faster than 2000 words per minute, the boy guessed most of the text just as a high-school pupil does when reading at the rate of 500-600 words per minute. The records of the eye movements of this boy during reading were the most unusual of any Taylor observed during his investigation of about 10,000 subjects. In the course of one fixation the boy perceived several words or even a whole phrase. Taylor emphasizes that this young reader was very gifted. At the age of 20 years he obtained a doctoral degree and soon after became a teacher at one of the leading universities.

Reading speed is determined not by the properties of the muscular apparatus of the eyes, but by the capacity and the special features of the individual's higher nervous activity. For this reason, when teaching pupils to read, attention should be concentrated on the accuracy with which the student reads and not on increasing the speed of his reading. The necessary speed will appear without special training, and usually at the end of his studies the pupil will be able to grasp the material in accordance with his capabilities.

3. ROLE OF EYE MOVEMENTS IN ASSESSING SPATIAL RELATIONSHIPS

Let us now consider a series of experiments showing the role of eye movements when the observer needs to assess proportions and to compare lengths, areas, and angles.

In one experiment in which a bright after-image, rectangular in shape, was created for a subject by means of a flashing light in a totally dark room, the subject was told to determine the ratio between

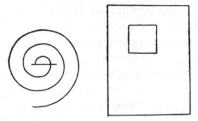

Fig. 126. Drawings for solving certain visual problems mentioned in the text.

the sides of this rectangle.   Although this task seems simple at first glance, it was really quite complicated because the subject could not use his eye movements for comparing the size of the rectangle. The subject's records show that the attempt to discover the ratio between the sides was accompanied by rotation of the eyes, the head, and even of the trunk (sometimes, when turning the trunk, the subject turned the chair on which he sat).   After these attempts had proved unsuccessful, the subject decided to attack the problem by means of complicated calculations.   This second method of solution appeared much more complicated than the method using eye movements.

For some idea of the two ways of solving problems analogous to that just mentioned, look at Fig. 126. On the left, a spiral and a short horizontal straight line are seen.   The problem is to determine the length of the spiral using the straight line as a unit of measurement. This problem is relatively easily solved with the use of eye movements (applying the unit of measurement along the spiral).   If, on the other hand, the center of the spiral is fixated, continuously and the subject meanwhile attempts to determine its length visually, the problem becomes very complex, although during fixation the whole spiral and the horizontal line are clearly and simultaneously visible to the observer.   On the right in Fig. 126 is a drawing of a rectangle and a small square by means of which the reader is instructed to measure the area of the rectangle.   Again, it is clear that the problem becomes very complex if one tries to solve it under conditions of continuous fixation; if eye movements can be used, however, the problem is relatively simple.   Much may be learned from problems such as these (problems in two and three dimensions).

A curious experiment was carried out by means of the P_4 cap (see the description of the cap).   The cap was affixed to one eye, and the second eye was covered with a bandage.   The reader will remember that the perception of surrounding objects through such a cap placed the observer in a situation in which he saw objects perfectly clearly but could not use eye movements at will.   For example, a change by the subject from a visible point of fixation A to a point B visible by the periphery of the retina always had the result that, after a saccade, a certain point C became fixed, situated at a distance from point A which might be twice as great as the distance AB. Examination of objects, photographs, and drawings through the P_4 cap led, the subject reported, to chaotic (out of control and unpredictable) movement of the object examined. Although the objects were seen clearly and were clearly recognized by the subject, problems such as those illustrated in Fig. 126 either could not be solved or were solved with considerable difficulty. The observer felt helpless and experienced an unpleasant sensation. When in these conditions the pursuit system of the eyes was put into operation involuntarily (and then not stopped until the end of the experiment) and the whole visible world acquired an oscillatory movement (usually the optical axis of the eye moved over the surface of a cone), the subject almost lost his bearings.

The statement that the subject clearly recognized objects in the experiment with the P_4 cap means that he saw and recognized without distortion peoples' faces, complex drawings, and even optical illusions.

This section may be summarized as follows. Micromovements of the eyes (drifts, small saccades) are necessary to maintain the high resolving power of the eye. It does not matter whether the micromovements of the eyes and of the retinal image are in harmony (as with the use of the P_4 cap) or not. All that matters is that the magnitude of the micromovement of the eye and that of the retinal image remain approximately the same. In either case, the resolving power of the eye at the moment of fixation of attention is the same, and there is no difference in the perception of fixated objects.

Macromovements of the eyes (large saccades) are necessary usually for the solution of certain problems (visual assessment of proportion, and length, comparison of areas and angles, etc.). Many visual assessments are invariably accompanied by macromovements. The solution of particular problems is always accompanied by certain movements. This association is so stable, and its role is so important, that many visual assessments would be almost impossible without macromovements of the eyes. If a subject does manage to solve such a problem without macromovements of the eyes, much more time is required to do so and the solution is always less accurate.

4. OPTICAL ILLUSIONS AND EYE MOVEMENTS

Several authors have tried to explain the appearance of well known optical illusions by movements of the eyes. It was interesting to ascertain whether these illusions persisted when the subject could not use eye movements during perception (i.e., when the subject looked at drawings evoking illusions through the P_4 cap). The subject was shown drawings that usually evoked illusions in the assessment of distances between the edges of objects, illusions that a segment of a straight line was displaced or deformed, etc.   It was found that all the illusions persisted; consequently, they cannot be attributed to eye movements.

Subsequent experiments showed that optical illusions also were preserved when the retinal image was strictly stationary relative to the retina.   This fact was investigated by means of a flashing light illuminating illusive drawings in a darkned room. The duration of the flashes was about 0.001 sec; the retinal image could therefore be regarded as

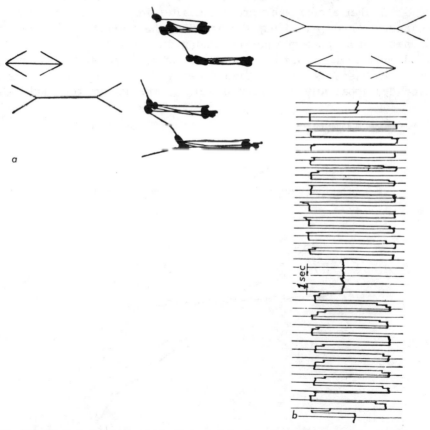

Fig. 127. Optical illusion: both horizontal lines are of equal length. Records of eye movements accompanying comparison of length.   a) On stationary photographic paper; b) made with photokymograph.

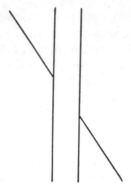

Fig. 128. Illusion that segments of a straight line are displaced relative to each other.

practically stationary. At the same time the brightness of the flash was so great that a clear and prolonged after-image of the drawing appeared. When perceiving the drawing, the subject could judge the presence or absence of a corresponding illusion.

I pointed out earlier that even large saccades are often involuntary. In many cases, saccades, sometimes even a group or a series of saccades apparently voluntary in nature, are not entirely under the

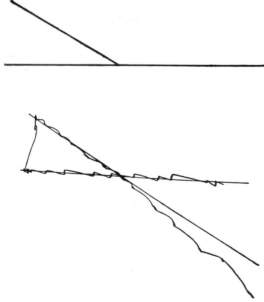

Fig. 129. Drawing and record of eye movements of a subject told to "follow with your eye the horizontal segments, then the sloping line, and continue the direction of the sloping line beyond the horizontal line."

observer's control.   This "disobedience" is particularly obvious in records of eye movements accompanying the perception of optical illusions.   A well known illusion arising in the assessment of distances between the edges of objects and a record of the eye movements accompanying the assessment of the drawing are shown in Fig. 127. It is clear from this figure that saccades of different amplitude correspond to objectively equal segments.   Here the visual evaluation of length and the amplitude of the saccades are in mutual agreement.

Many experiments such as that illustrated in Fig. 127 show that the subject's subjective evaluation may always be judged from the eye movements made during comparison of distances.   Subjective evaluation of distance in many cases depends on the shape and position of the objects the distance between which is being assessed.   At first glance this may appear strange, but, for example, objectively equal distances between two vertical lines and two ends of a horizontal line are assessed differently.   The length of a horizontal line appears much less to some observers than the distance between the vertical lines, and this difference is reflected in the eye-movement records.

Since illusions similar to those illustrated in Fig. 127 continue to occur both in experiments with the P_4 cap and with a stationary retinal image, when the drawing is illuminated by a flashing light, we may conclude that eye movement has no appreciable effect on the presence of many illusions. On the other hand, as the records show, the presence of illusions appreciably influences the amplitude of the saccades accompanying the evaluation of distances.

Let us consider another example. The familiar illusion of displaced segments of a straight line is shown in Fig. 128.   The record shown in Fig. 129 illustrates that during the visual extension of a straight line, the observer slightly changes its direction, increasing the angle between

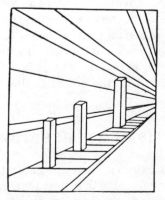

Fig. 130. Illusion of perspective.

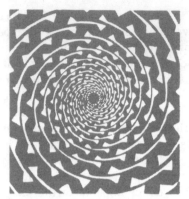

Fig. 131. The deceptive spiral.

the prolonged straight line and the intersecting line. As in the previous case, this and similar illusions are nor due to the movements of the eyes, but themselves bring about a change in the direction of visual pursuit.

I have given only two cases demonstrating how optical illusions may influence eye movements. Many types of optical illusions are now known. Some of these are easily explained, for example, illusions of a change in the apparent size of objects depending on their brightness (we see bright objects bigger than dark objects of the same size). Such illusions are due to an effect of irradiation (Kravkov, 1950). Some illusions have a definitely central origin, and these also are easily explained. The origin of many illusions is not yet known, however; the explanations advanced to date cannot be regarded as convincing. Different illusions influence eye movements to different degrees and in different ways. At the same time, some optical illusions have no influence whatever on eye movements. As an example of this last case, the reader should carefully consider the two strong illusions illustrated in Figs. 130 and 131. For instance, the illusion in Fig. 130 has no effect on the movements of the eyes, but if an observer attempts to follow the outline of the deceptive spiral in Fig. 131 with his eye, it will frequently jump from one turn of the spiral to the next.

5. EYE MOVEMENTS AND PERCEPTION OF MOVEMENTS

When we look at stationary objects around us, every shift of the points of fixation is accompanied by a displacement of the retinal image over the retina. Although the perception of surrounding objects is constantly accompanied by these displacements of the retinal image, we see all stationary objects as stationary. On the other hand, when a moving object appears in the field of vision of our eyes, the movement of its image over the retina is such that moving objects are seen as moving. Then, under conditions of pursuit, (when the retinal image is slightly mobile relative to the retina), the eye continues to see it as a moving object.

Comparison of these two facts shows that types of retinal-image and eye movements exist during which, in accordance with objective reality, perceived objects appear to us to be moving, and that types of retinal-image and eye movements exist during which perceived objects appear to us to be stationary. Let us try to determine the combinations of eye and retinal-image movements (or immobility) with which objects are seen as moving and the combinations with which they are seen as stationary.

As a result of a saccade, and synchronously with it, the retinal image of a stationary object moves across the retina through an angle equal to the angle of rotation of the eye, in a direction directly opposite to the direction of movement of the retina. The visual object is then seen as stationary, and a large enough saccade is always perceived as a change of the points of fixation (transfer of attention) on a stationary object. In some experiments with the P_4 cap, the retinal image of the object moved in step with the saccades in a given direction so that the angle of rotation of the eye and the angle of displacement of the retinal image always differed in magnitude, and the direction of the displacement of the retinal image was directly opposite to the direction of movement of the retina, as under normal conditions. In this case, the visual object always appeared to the subject to be moving jerkily. Naturally, the smaller this difference, the smaller the movement of the object appeared to be; when the difference became on the order of involuntary saccades during fixation (5-15 minutes of angle), the object appeared to the subject to be stationary. If the direction of the retinal-image shift in step with the saccade was not directly opposite to the direction of movement of the retina, the visual object also appeared to the subject to be moving jerkily.

Some particularly interesting experiments have been carried out in which a visual object occupying a comparatively small part of the visual field remained stationary relative to the retina at the moment of a saccade (or any other eye movement) and at the moment of rest. Such conditions may be regarded as an ideal which the system of pursuit strives to reach, although it never succeeds. P_7 and P_8 caps were used in the experiments. The test field, stationary relative to the retina, was, in some experiments, a transparent shadow visible to the subject against the background of surrounding stationary objects. In some experiments the stationary test field was an opaque shutter, also seen by the subject against a background of stationary checkered objects. These experiments showed that any test field, stationary relative to the retina, visible to an observer against the background of stationary objects, appears to be moving during movements of the eye, and these movements coincide in direction and velocity with the movements of the eye. In this case the perception of movement of the object is preserved even when an active system of pursuit is no longer needed, and either has ceased to work or is idling.

If the eye is at rest, movement of the retinal image, not too fast and not too slow, over the retina is always perceived by the subject as movement of the object. We see moving objects as moving not only when we pursue them, but also when our attention is stationary. This conclusion is valid even when the retinal image of an object moves against an empty field occupying the whole field of vision (as in the experiments with "comets" and other experiments in Chapter II).

In a series of experiments using the P_4 cap, holes were made in the cap mirror so that the subject's field of vision appeared to be split into two different parts (one field will appear inside the other). The visual objects in the part of the visual field perceived by means of the mirror were in a state of constant and irregular movement, for the subject could not choose his points of fixation at will, and his attempt to do so led to the result mentioned earlier. In the second (smaller) part of the field of vision (corresponding to the hole in the mirror), perception was as usual and the subject could use eye movements at will. Since the second (inner) field of vision was surrounded by a field in which everything was moving about at random, the question arose whether or not these surroundings influence the perception of objects visible through the hole in the mirror of the cap.

The experiments showed that when the fields were related in a certain way, when the outer field was large enough and the inner field small enough, some influence of the surroundings was observed. The objects in the inner field appeared displaced towards the side opposite to the apparent movement of the objects in the outer field.

This fact suggests that the evaluation of the whole situation in which a person finds himself in each concrete case plays a role in the evaluation of the mobility or immobility of surrounding objects. Mistakes in the evaluation of mobility and immobility of surrounding objects are observed in many pathological cases. Such disturbances may be caused by a discrepancy between the muscular effort and the actual movement of the eyes. By interfering with the free movement of the eye or by exerting pressure upon it, we may observe an apparent displacement of visual objects.

In conclusion, we repeat once again that under normal conditions, with the head stationary and under ordinary conditions of perception, an object appears stationary to us first, if the eye and the retinal image of the object are simultaneously stationary (the process of fixation on a stationary object) or if the retinal image of the object, synchronously with the eye movement during a saccade, moves relative to the retina through the angle of rotation of the eye with the angular velocity of the eye in a direction directly opposite to the retinal movement. In all other cases, the observer sees the object as moving in the visual field. An object is also seen as moving when the eye is stationary, but the retinal image is moving over the retina, and also when the retinal image is stationary (and seen against a background of stationary objects), but the eye is moving.

6. ROLE OF RECOGNITION IN EVALUATION OF SPATIAL RELATIONSHIPS

The perception of surrounding objects, the evaluation of distances, and the determination of the relative arrangement of objects are accompanied not only by eye movements, but also by rotation of the head function of the vestibular apparatus, and the use of all our ontogenetic experience towards constancy of perception and recognition.

It is evident that during examination of objects turns of the head play the same role as eye movements. The immobility of the surrounding objects apparent to an observer when he turns his head is maintained in perception by the vestibular apparatus. In this section I would emphasize that recognition also plays an important role in evaluation of the spatial arrangement of surrounding objects. The following case is an instructive illustration of this.

Near a small wood, on the bank of one of the Volga reservoirs, an old wooden barge was moored against the bank to serve as a landing stage. A little two-room house had been built on the barge; an elderly couple (employed by the river steamship line) lived there in the summertime and worked on the landing stage. The landing stage was a busy place. The house and its surroundings were very familiar to many visitors. One day, however, the water level in the reservoir fell by almost a meter and a half below the normal level. The barge, one end of which rested on the bank, sloped steeply when the water level fell, approximately by 15°. Naturally the house on the barge, and everything in it, sloped at the same angle. The perception of anyone who, when walking along the sloping surface of the barge, glanced or walked through the open door of the house was very interesting. The furniture and other things in both rooms had been fastened in their old places, so that everything appeared as usual. Every visitor looking into the room involuntarily placed his body in the position perpendicular to the floor of the house (i.e., at an angle of approximately 75° to the horizontal); he would either fall to the ground or land on one of the walls of the room, which he would hold on to for some time until he regained his balance, and began to move about the room unsteadily, holding on to the walls and furniture.

The view from the window of the little house, if part of the room, or at least the window frame, were included within the field of vision, was quite fantastic. The horizon, the surface of the water, and the surrounding neighborhood were all seen as sloping. Moreover, the large Volga steamers were plying on this sloping surface of the water, themselves at an improbable angle.

There was a telephone in one room. When speaking on the telephone, the visitors usually overcame their unsteadiness and stood with body vertical. To another visitor sitting at the table, the position of a person speaking on the telephone appeared completely unnatural and very funny. It was quite incomprehensible how he managed to stand on his feet when his body was inclined to such a degree. A body moving upright in these conditions looked like a circus trick. Many other details were equally unnatural. For example, it was amusing to see the line of tea in a cup or the weights of the clock, which some-how seemed to have come away from the wall and to be hanging in space because of mysterious forces.

This example illustrates the important role of recognition of a situation as a whole in our perception. By recognizing a familiar environment and using this as a basis, we thereby evaluate all the secondary elements of what we see. If we are mistaken in the evalua-tion of our basis, the second-degree elements may appear distorted to us, and as our example shows, these distortions remain even if they are contrary to common sense and to the indications of the vestibular apparatuṣ.

This example suggests that what is in general a very important and desirable feature of our perception may lead under certain unusual and rare conditions to distortion, or in other words, to optical illusions. An illusion of this type was shown in Fig. 130. Here we recognize and see a road going into the distance, and columns standing at the edge of the road. In natural conditions in accordance with the laws of perspective, the size of the retinal image of the columns should diminish with an increasing distance from the observer (if all the columns objectively are of the same height). If, on the other hand, the retinal images of the columns at different distances from the observer are equal, the columns are in fact of different sizes. This is the case we recognize in Fig. 130, so that the objectively equal columns in the drawing appear to be different sizes.

CONCLUSIONS

The human eyes voluntarily and involuntarily fixate on those elements of an object which carry or may carry essential and useful information. The more information is contained in an element, the longer the eyes stay on it. The distribution of points of fixation on the object changes depending on the purpose of the observer, i.e., depending on the information which he must obtain, for different information can usually be obtained from different parts of an object. The order and duration of the fixations on elements of an object are determined by the thought process accompanying the analysis of the information obtained. Hence people who think differently also, to some extent, see differently.

Normally, reading speed depends not on the muscular apparatus of a person's eyes, but on his higher nervous activity.

Optimal conditions for the solution of certain problems (visual evaluation of proportions, estimation of length, comparison of areas, angles, and so on) require macromovements of the eyes (large saccades). Without these, many visual evaluations are impossible or attended by great difficulty and considerable waste of time.

In ordinary conditions of perception, an object is seen as stationary: first, if the eye and the retinal image of the object are stationary (the process of fixation on a stationary object); second, if, synchronously with the movement during a saccade, the retinal image of the object moves relative to the retina through the angle of rotation of the eye with the angular velocity of the eye, in a direction opposite to the retinal movement. In all other cases, the observer sees the object as moving in the field of vision. Specifically, an object is seen as moving: first, when the eye is stationary, but the retinal image moves over the retina; and second, when the retinal image is stationary (and is seen by the observer against the background of stationary objects), but the eye is moving.

LITERATURE CITED

Adamson, J. Ocular scanning and depth perception, Nature 168(4269):345 (1951).
Adler, F.H., and Fliegelman, M. Arch. Ophthalm. 12:475 (1934).
Adrian, E.D. The Basis of Sensations, London, 1928.
Averbakh, M.I. Ophthalmological Sketches, Moscow—Leningrad, 1940.
Barlow, H.B. Eye movements during fixation, J. Physiol. (Engl.) 116(3):209 (1952).
Boeck, W. Die Physiologie der Augenbewegungen, Deutsche Opt. Wochenschr. 6:48 (1951).
Bongard, M.M., and Smirnov, M.S. Doklady Akad. Nauk SSSR 102(6):1111 (1955).
Buswell, G.T. How adults read, Suppl. Educ. Mongr. (45), Chicago, 1937.
Byford, G.H. Eye movement recording, Nature 184(suppl. 19):1493 (1959).
Carmichael, L., and Dearborn, W.F. Reading and Visual Fatigue, London, 1948.
Clark, B.C. Amer. J. Psychol. 46:325 (1934).
Clarke, F.J. Optica Acta (7):219 (1960).
Clowes, M.B. Some factors in brightness discrimination with constraint of retinal image movement, Optica Acta 8(1):61 (1961).
Clowes, M.B., and Ditchburn, R.W. An improved apparatus for producing a stabilized retinal image, Optica Acta 6(3):252 (1959).
Cobb, P.W., and Moss, F,K. J. Franklin Inst. 200:239 (1925).
Cords, R. Graefes Arch. Ophthal. 118:771 (1927)
Cornsweet, T.N. New technique for the measurement of small eye movements, J. Opt. Soc. Amer. 49(11):808 (1958).
Crawford, W.A. Visual accuity, eye movements, and head-eye movement integration, J. Physiol. (Engl.) 145(2):50 (1959).
Delabarre, E.B. Amer. J. Psychol. 9:572 (1898).
Ditchburn, R.W. Problems of visual discrimination, 20th Thomas Young oration, delivered to the society November 12, 1959.
Ditchburn, R.W. Eye movements in relation to perception of color, Visual Problems Colour 2:51 (1961).
Ditchburn, R.W., and Fender, D.H. The stabilized retinal image, Optica Acta 2(3):128 (1955).
Ditchburn, R.W., Fender, D.H., and Mayne, S. Vision with controlled movements of the retinal image, J. Physiol. (Engl.) 145:98 (1959).
Ditchburn, R.W., and Ginsborg, B.L. Vision with a stabilized retinal image, Nature 170 (4314):36 (1952).
Ditchburn, R.W., and Ginsborg, B.L. Involuntary eye movements during fixation, J. Physiol. (Engl.) 119(1):1 (1953).
Ditchburn, R.W., and Pritchard, R.M. Binocular vision with two stabilized retinal images, Quart. J. Exp. Psychol. 12(1):26 (1960).
Dodge, R. Psychol. Monogr. 8(4), 1907.
Dodge, R., and Cline, T.S. Psychol. Rev. 8:145 (1901).
Dohlman, G. Acta Oto-Laryng. Suppl. 5:78 (1925).
Dohlman, G. Acta Oto-Laryng. Suppl. 23:50 (1935).
Drischel, H., and Lange. Über den Frequenzgang der horizontalen Folgebewegungen des menschlichen Auges, Pflüger's Arch. Ges. Physiol. 262(4):307-333 (1956).
Drischel, H., Pflüger's Arch. Ges. Physiol. 262(1):34 (1958).

Duke-Elder, W.S. Textbook of Ophthalmology, Vol. 1, London, 1932.

Fender, D.H., and Mayne, S. Visibility of a fine line in intermittent illumination, Optica Acta 7(2):129 (1960).

Fender, D.H., and Nye, P.W. An investigation of the mechanisms of eye movement control, Kibernetic 1(2):81 (1961).

Ford, A., White, C.T., and Lichtenstein, M. Analysis of eye movements during free search, J. Opt. Soc. Amer. 49(3):287 (1959).

Fulton, J.E. Physiology of the Nervous System, Oxford, 1943.

Gaarder, K. Relating a component of physiological nystagmus to visual display, Science 132(3425):471 (1960).

Gassovskii, L.N., and Nikol'skaya, N.A. Mobility of the eye during fixation, Problemy Fiziol. Optiki 1:173 (1941).

George, E.J., Toren, J.A., and Lowell, J.W. Amer. J. Ophthal. 6:833 (1923).

Gilbert, L.C. Functional Motor Efficiency of the Eyes and Its Relation to Reading, Vol. 11, Univ. of California Press, Berkeley—Los Angeles, 1953, p. 159.

Ginsborg, B.L. Rotation of the eyes during involuntary blinking, Nature 169(4297):412 (1952).

Glezer, V.D. Role of convergence in stereoscopic vision, Biofizika 4(3):329 (1959).

Glezer, V.D., and Tsukkerman, I.I. Information and Vision, Izd-vo AN SSSR, Moscow—Leningrad, 1961.

Granit, R. The Electrophysiological Investigation of Reception (Russian translation), IL, 1957.

Gregory, R.L. Eye movements and the stability of the visual world, Nature 182(4644):1214 (1958).

Gurevich, B. Kh. Orientation of the eye on the basis of muscle sense and the possible role of proprioception in visual fixation, Doklady Akad. Nauk SSSR 115(4):829 (1957).

Gurevich, B. Kh. The universal characteristics of fixation saccades of the eye, Biofizika 6(3):377 (1961).

Haberich, F.I., and Fischer, M.H. Die Bedeutung des Lidschlags für das Sehen beim Umherblicken, Pflüger's Arch. Ges. Physiol. 267(6):626 (1958).

Hartridge, H. The visual perception of fine detail, Philos. Trans. Roy. Soc. London B 232:592 (1947).

Hartridge, H., and Thomson, L.C. Methods of investigating eye movements, Brit. J. Ophthalm. 32(9):581 (1948).

Helmholtz, H. Physiol. Optics 3, 1925.

Higgins and Stultz, K.F. Frequency and amplitude of ocular tremor, J. Opt. Soc. Amer. 43(12):1136 (1953).

Hodgson, F., and Lord, M.P. Measurement of eye movements accompanying voluntary head movements, Nature 174(4419):75 (1954).

Holmes, G. Brit. J. Ophthalm. 2, 1918.

Huey, E.B. Amer. J. Psychol. 9:575 (1898).

Huey, E.B. Amer. J. Psychol. 11:283 (1900).

Hyde, I.D. Some characteristics of voluntary human ocular movements in the horizontal plane, Amer. J. Ophthalm. 48:85 (1959).

Illig, H., Pelanz, M., and Uexküll, T. von. Experimentelle Untersuchungen über die kleinste Zeiteinheit (Moment) der optischen Wahrnehmung, Pflüger's Arch. Ges. Physiol. 257(2):121 (1953).

Jacobson, E. Amer. J. Physiol. 91:567 (1930).

Jacobson, E. Amer. J. Physiol. 95:694 (1930).

Javal, L.E. Ann. Oculist. 82:242 (1879).

Jones, L.A., and Higgins, G.C. J. Opt. Soc. Amer. 37:217 (1947).

Judd, C.H., McAllister, C.N., and Steele, W.M. Psychol. Monogr. 7(1), 1905.

Karslake, J.S. J. Appl. Psychol. 24:417 (1940).

Keesey, U.T. Effects of involuntary eye movements on visual acuity, J. Opt. Soc. Amer. 50(8):769 (1960).

Knoll, H.A. Research with tilting haploscope, J. Opt. Soc. Amer. 49(12):1176 (1959).

Krauskopf, J. Effect of retinal image motion on contrast thresholds for maintaining vision, J. Opt. Soc. Amer. 47(8):740 (1957).

Krauskopf, J., Cornsweet, T.N., and Riggs, L.A. Analysis of eye movements during monocular and binocular fixation, J. Opt. Soc. Amer. 50(6):572 (1960).

Kravkov, S.V. The Eye and Its Work, Izd-vo AN SSSR, Moscow—Leningrad, 1950.

Kravkov, S.V. Color Vision, Izd-vo AN SSSR, Moscow—Leningrad, 1951.

Lamansky, S. Pflüger's Arch. Ges. Physiol. 2:418 (1869).

Lancaster, W.B. Amer. J. Ophthalm. 24:485 (1941).

Landolt, A. Arch. d'Ophthalm. 11:385 (1891).

Lion, K.S., and Powsner, E.R. An ergographic method for testing ocular muscles, J. Appl. Physiol. 4:276 (1951).

Lord, M.P. Proc. Phys. Soc. 61:489 (1948).

Lord, M.P. Measurement of binocular eye movements of subjects, Ophthalmologica 35(1-2):21 (1951).

Lord, M.P. Eye rotations with changes of accommodation, Nature 170(4329):670 (1952a).

Lord, M.P. Binocular eye movements when convergence is subjectively changed, Nature 169(4311):1011 (1952b).

Lord, M.P., and Wright, W.D. Eye movements during monocular fixation, Nature 162(4105):25 (1948).

Lord, M.P., and Wright, W.D. Nature 163:803 (1949).

Lord, M.P., and Wright, W.D. The investigation of eye movements, Reports on Progress in Physics 13(1):23 (1950).

Loring, M.W. Psychol. Rev. 22:354 (1915).

Luriya, A.R., Pravdina-Vinarskaya, E.N., and Yarbus, A.L. Mechanisms of eye movements in the process of visual perception and their pathology, Voprosy Psikhologii No. 5, p. 160, 1961.

Mackworth, N.F., and Mackworth, H.H. Eye fixations recorded on changing visual scenes by the television eye-marker, J. Opt. Soc. Amer. 48(7):439 (1958).

Marx, E., and Trendelenburg, W. Sinnesphysiol. 45:87 (1911).

Meyers, I.L. Arch. Neurol. Psychiat. 21:901 (1929).

Miles, W.R. Science 90:404 (1939a).

Miles, W.R. Yale J. Biol. Med. 12:161 (1939b).

Miles, W.R. Science 91:456 (1940).

Miller, J.W., and Ludvigh, E. The perception of movement persistence in the Ganzfeld, J. Opt. Soc. Amer. 51(1):57 (1961).

Monnier, M., and Hufshmidt, II.J. Helv. Physiol. Pharmacol. Acta 8(2):30 (1950).

Mowrer, O.H., Ruch, T.C., and Miller, N.E. Amer. J. Physiol. 114:423 (1936).

Müller, J. Zur vergleichenden Physiologie des Gesichtssinnes des Menschen und der Thiere. Nebst einem Versuch über die Bewegungen der Augen und über den menschlichen Blick, Cnobloch, Leipzig, 1826, p. 251.

Nachmias, J. Two-dimensional motion of the retinal image during monocular fixation, J. Opt. Soc. Amer. 49(9):901 (1959).

Nachmias, J. Meridional variations in visual acuity and eye movements during fixation, J. Opt. Soc. Amer. 50(6):569 (1960).

Newhall, S.N. Amer. J. Psychol. 40:628 (1928).

Oesterberg, G. Topography of Layer of Rods and Cones in the Human Retina, Copenhagen, 1935.

Ogle, K.N. The role of convergence in stereoscopic vision, Proc. Phys. Soc. B 66(402):513 (1953).

Ogle, K.N., Mussey, F., and Prangen, A. Amer. J. Ophthalm. 32:1069 (1949).

Ohm, J. Augenheilk. 32:4 (1914).

Ohm, J. Augenheilk. 36:198 (1916).

Ohm, J. Graefes Arch. Ophthalm. 120:235 (1928).

Orschansky, I. Z. Physiol. 12:785 (1899).

Park, G.E. Arch. Ophthalm. 15:703 (1936a).

Park, G.E. J. Ophthalm. 19:967 (1936b).

Park, G.E., and Park, R. Amer. J. Physiol. 104:545 (1933).

Park, G.E., and Park, R. Arch. Ophthalm. 23:1216 (1940).

Peckham, R.H. Arch. Ophthalm. 12:562 (1934).

Pivotti, G., and Lucarelli, A. Contributo al moderni metodi di registrazione nistagmografica, Boll. Soc. Ital. Biol. Sperim. 31(3/4):267 (1955).

Polyak, S. The Retina, Chicago, 1941.

Rashbass, C. Barbiturate nystagmus and the mechanism of visual fixation, Nature 183(4665): 897 (1959).

Rashbass, C. The relationship between saccadic and smooth tracking eye movements, J. Physiol. (Engl.) 159(2):326 (1961).

Rashbass, C., and Westheimer, G. Disjunctive eye movements, J. Physiol. (France) 159:339 (1961).

Rashbass, C., and Westheimer, G. Independence of conjugate and disjunctive eye movements, J. Physiol. (Engl.) 159(2):361 (1961).

Ratliff, F.A., and Riggs, L.A. Involuntary motions of the eye during monocular fixation, J. Exp. Psychol. 40(6):687 (1950).

Riggs, L.A., and Niehl, E.W. Eye movements recorded during convergence and divergence, J. Opt. Soc. Amer. 50(9):913 (1960).

Riggs, L.A., and Ratliff, F. Visual acuity and the normal tremor of the eyes, Science 114(2949):17 (1951).

Riggs, L.A., Armington, J.C., and Ratliff, F. Motions of the retinal image during fixation, J. Opt. Soc. Amer. 44(4):315 (1954).

Riggs, L.A., Ratliff, F., Cornsweet, J.C., and Cornsweet, T.N. The disappearance of steadily fixated visual test objects, J. Opt. Soc. Amer. 43(6):495 (1953).

Schott, E. Deut. Arch. Klin. Med. 140:79 (1922).

Shackel, B. Note on mobile eye viewpoint recording, J. Opt. Soc. Amer. 50(8):763 (1960).

Shakhnovich, A.R. and V.R. Pupillographia, Publ.-Medicine, Moscow, 1961.

Shortess, G.K. Role of involuntary eye movements in stereoscopic acuity, J. Opt. Soc. Amer. 51:555 (1961).

Smith, W.M., and Warter, P.J. Photoelectric technique for measuring eye movements, Science 130(3384):1248 (1959).

Smith, W.M., and Warter, P.J. Eye movement and stimulus movement; new photoelectric electromechanical system for recording and measuring tracking motions of the eye, J. Opt. Soc. Amer. 50(3):245 (1960).

Stigler, R. Das Kinesimeter. Ein Apparat zur Bestimmung des optischen Wahrnehmungs-vermögens für kleinste Bewegungen, 104(2):116 (1951).

Stratton, G.M. Phil. Stud. 20:336 (1902).

Stratton, G.M. Psychol. Rev. 13:8 (1906).

Taylor, E.A. Controlled Reading, Chicago, 1937.

Taylor, E.A. The spans: perception, apprehension, and recognition as related to reading and speed reading, Amer. J. Ophthalm. 44(4):501 (1957).

Tinker, M.A. Amer. J. Psychol. 43:115 (1931).

Tonkov, V.N. A Textbook of Human Anatomy, Leningrad, 1946.

Vladimirov, A.D., and Khomskaya, E.D. A photoelectric method of recording eye movements, Voprosy Psikhologii (2):177 (1961).

Weaver, H.E. Psychol. Bull. 28:211 (1931).

Westheimer, G. A note on the response characteristics of the extraocular muscle system, Bull. Math. Biophys. 20:149 (1958).

Yarbus, A.L. Some illusions in the evaluation of apparent distances between edges of objects, in: Investigations of the Psychology of Perception, Izd-vo AN SSSR, Moscow, 1948.

Yarbus, A.L. Some illusions in the evaluation of apparent parts and sums of segments of distances, Problemy Fiziol. Optiki 9, 1950.

Yarbus, A.L. Overestimation of the top portion of a figure, Problemy Fiziol. Optiki 10, 1952.

Yarbus, A.L. Investigation of the principles governing eye movements in the process of vision, Doklady Akad. Nauk SSSR 96(4):732 (1954).

Yarbus, A.L. Eye movements during change in points of fixation, Trudy Inst. Biol. Fiziki 1, 1955a.

Yarbus, A.L. Eye movements in rod monochromats, Trudy Inst. Biol. Fiziki 1, 1955b.

Yarbus, A.L. Recording eye movements during reading and examinations of pictures on flat surfaces, in: Collection in Memory of Academician P.P. Lazarev, Izd-vo AN SSSR, Moscow, 1956a.

Yarbus, A.L. The visual assessment of distances, in: Collection in Memory of Academician P.P. Lazarev, Izd-vo AN SSSR, Moscow, 1956b.

Yarbus, A.L. Eye movements during change in points of fixation, Biofizika 1(1):76 (1956c).

Yarbus, A.L. The plethysmogram of the eye, Biofizika 1(3):242 (1956d).

Yarbus, A.L. Perception of the stationary retinal image, Biofizika 1(5):435 (1956e).

Yarbus, A.L. Velocity of movement of the image of a stationary point on the retina during fixation, Biofizika 1(6):593 (1956f).

Yarbus, A.L. A new method of recording eye movements, Biofizika 1(8):713 (1956g).

Yarbus, A.L. A new technique of investigating the function of various parts of the retina, Biofizika 2(2):163 (1957a).

Yarbus, A.L. Eye movements during a change in stationary points of fixation in space, Biofizika 2(6):698 (1957b).

Yarbus, A.L. Perception of an image stationary relative to the retina, Biofizika 2(6):703 (1957c).

Yarbus, A.L. Perception of images moving across the retina at a given speed, Biofizika 4(3):320 (1959a).

Yarbus, A.L. The role of eye movements in the process of vision, Biofizika 4(6):757 (1959b).

Yarbus, A.L. Perception of images of variable luminance, stationary relative to the retina, Biofizika 5(2):158 (1960a).

Yarbus, A.L. Perception of images of great luminance, stationary relative to the retina, Biofizika 5(3):293 (1960b).

Yarbus, A.L. Eye movements during examination of complex objects, Biofizika 6(2):207 (1961).

Yarbus, A.L. Eye movements during perception of moving objects, Biofizika 7(1):64 (1962a).

Yarbus, A.L. Some experiments with an image stationary relative to the retina, Biofizika 7(2):207 (1962b).

Yarbus, A.L. Perception of images of changing color stationary relative to the retina, Biofizika 7(3):333 (1962c).

Yarbus, A.L. The perception of flickering images stationary relative to the retina, Biofizika 7(5):615 (1962d).

Yarbus, A.L., and Gol'tsman, N. Movements of the eyes during perception of images in stereoscopic motion pictures, Trudy Inst. Biol. Fiziki 1, 1955.

Zinchenko, V.P. Eye movements and formation of an image, Voprosy Psikhologii No. 5, 1958.

INDEX